PERSONALIZED WEIGHT TRAINING FOR FITNESS AND ATHLETICS

From Theory to Practice

Frederick C. Hatfield, Ph.D.
University of Wisconsin

March L. Krotee, Ph.D.
University of Minnesota

D1276628

KENDALL/HUNT PUBLISHING COMPANY
2460 Kerper Boulevard, Dubuque, Iowa 52001

B   401830   02

Contents

Preface

Upon reviewing the many texts and articles on the general subjects of weight training, weight lifting, strength fitness, conditioning or exercise programs, we have encountered one basic problem. While most texts offer a relatively complete overview of the field, none are arranged so that easy transfer from theoretical to practical aspects of training is accomplished. The student is not led in any clear, meaningful fashion from the physiological mechanisms underlying training technique to actual practice of them. All too frequently, random bits of physiological data are presented, usually serving to confuse the student further as to the "whys" and "hows" of training. Why does one train with weights in a particular way to maximize power, endurance, or size, for example?

This text was devised on the thesis that it is no longer appropriate or desirable simply to state that this is the way to do it. Students want to know why. By carefully selecting the most applicable physiological background information, this text leads into the principles and techniques underlying the "whys" and "hows" of weight training.

Another focal point of the text is the fact that much misinformation, generally in the form of gym gossip, is spread concerning the so-called dangers, good points, methods and systems of weight training. This text, although far from complete, attempts to dispel many of these myths and misunderstandings by introducing the scientific approach to training technique and regimen selection. Along this line, sections on proper training tables (diet), ergogenic aids, and beginners' through advanced students' regimen are provided. These sections are meant to serve as guidelines only, since every athlete or fitness enthusiast is confronted with problems which are largely personal. Therein lies the major contribution of the text—the personalized approach to training.

Another important contribution of the text is its applicability to women. Most texts on weight training either mention women's exercises in passing or fail to mention them at all. The approach used in this text is that women's training procedures and attendant physiological mechanisms are no different from those employed by men. The text is therefore applicable to both sexes.

Chapter 1 presents those physiological mechanisms which underlie one's choice of training regimen, while Chapters 2 and 3 deal specifically with the basic principles of training and systems of training, respectively. Chapter 4 presents an anatomical and practical approach to exercise selection and apparatus selection. Chapter 5 offers basic nutritional advice along with procedures for losing and gaining weight, as well as a section on ergogenic aids. Finally, Chapter 6 deals with training progress assessment and fitness assessment in an easily applied, unobtrusive sequence.

Traditionally covered topics such as Rx for elderly and rehabilitating persons, techniques of competitive weightlifting, calisthenics, and general training programs (nonpersonalized programs) are not included.

Acknowledgments

Many thanks are extended to the members of the Madison Weightlifting Center, and to the Center itself, for assisting in the production of this manuscript. A special note of thanks is extended to Dr. Ted Ritzer, Frank Gancarz, Floyd DeSpirito, and the very venerable coach Joe Mills, all of whom, at one time or another, patiently coached the first author in the finer points of strength development and competitive weight lifting. Deep gratitude is also extended to our wives, Mary and Leslie, respectively, for their encouragement and love.

Frederick C. Hatfield
March L. Krotee

Foreword

Interest in training with weights has accelerated in recent years as more and more persons discover the benefits of weightlifting.

In this publication the authors offer a clear and sensible approach to weight training. These easy-to-follow techniques are geared towards the athlete, the fitness enthusiast, the body builder. Its program can be followed by both men and women.

The authors begin with a presentation of the major theoretical concepts of weight training, then establish scientific precedence for training methods.

Their explanation of the exercises is kinesiologically accurate and easily understood, augmented by ample illustrations.

The authors' technique for measuring your own personal progress is invaluable, and their outline of weight control procedures and diets for competitors is excellent.

This work will serve as a boon to anyone with a desire for fitness and conditioning through weight training.

Sincerely,
Murray Levin
National Chairman
AAU Weightlifting Committee

Muscle Physiology

Contents: *Gross Muscle Structure*
Muscle Fiber Structure
Other Structural Considerations
Blood Supply to Muscle Fibers
Nerve Supply to Muscle Fibers
Energetics of Anaerobic and Aerobic Pathways
Mechanics of Muscular Contraction
Types of Muscle Fiber

1

Introduction

There is a marked tendency for people to embrace simplistic approaches to problems. Taking the path of least resistance may often lead to equitable solutions and answers, but there are also instances that require relatively complex background information and understandings. Such is the case in weight training and conditioning. However, lest the reader immediately become turned off to the approach the present text espouses (there are many terms and phrases that are steeped in physiological jargon), it is the grasp of broad concepts that is important, not rote memorization of obscure facts. The reader is invited to become familiar with the general principles of weight training through an understanding of the mechanisms of his/her physiology. While it is desirable for one to remember selected facts, it is not necessary. Further, the end result one should strive for is proficiency in devising training regimen that conforms to basic principles of exercise physiology, a task which requires a personalized approach.

Gross Muscle Structure

Picture the last time you prepared a thick steak for dinner. The white lines running through the meat are comprised of connective tissue called *perimysium*. The perimysium binds bundles of *fibers* together into a *fasciculus*. Each fiber is actually a muscle cell which has its own connective tissue—the *endomysium*. Binding all the fasciculii together is yet another sheath of connective tissue called the *epimysium*. This is the outermost covering of the gross musculature.

Each muscle fiber—that is, each individual cell—transmits its contractile force to these various connective tissues. Since the connective tissues are continuous with the muscle's *tendons,* the force is thereby transmitted to the bones to which the tendons connect, resulting in movement.

A muscle fiber can range in size from about .01 millimeter to .10 millimeter in diameter, and from about 1.00 millimeter to many millimeters in length. The size of a fiber generally depends upon the location of the muscle—that is, the function of the muscle. Gross movements generally improve muscles comprised of very long fibers, whereas fine movements such as ocular movements generally involve muscles with shorter fibers.

Along the same line of reasoning, muscles are differentiated according to their arrangement of muscle fibers. There are two general classifications of skeletal muscles: *fusiform* and *penniform*. Fusiform muscles' fibers are arranged parallel to the long axis of the muscle, and are either long or short. *Long fusiform* muscles are relatively weak but contract a great

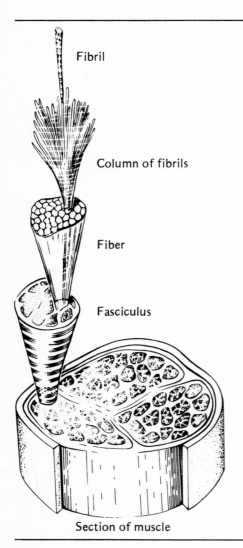

Fibril

Column of fibrils

Fiber

Fasciculus

Section of muscle

Figure 1-1. Construction of a section of muscle to show the relationship of its individual parts of the whole. An individual muscle fiber contains many fibrils, and a fasciculus contains many muscle fibers. A muscle is a composite of many fasciculi. Adapted from Sigmund Grollman's *The Human Body* Second Edition. Reprinted with permission of Macmillan Publishing Co., from *The Human Body* Second Edition by Sigmund Grollman. Copyright © 1969 by Sigmund Grollman.

distance. *Short fusiform* muscles are strong and have a very short contractile distance. Fusiform muscles are most commonly found in the extremities, although short fusiform muscles are found in the intercostal regions (i.e., between the ribs).

Penniform muscle fibers are arranged diagonally to the direction in which the muscle pulls. These muscles are found in the trunk as well as in the extremities. Because of the diagonal arrangement of the fibers, they do not contract over as great a distance as the fusiform muscles do, but are much stronger. There are three different classifications of penniform muscles: *unipennate,* with the fibers arranged on one side of the tendon; *bipennate,* with the fibers arranged on both sides of the tendon; and *multipennate,* with fibers attaching to several tendons.

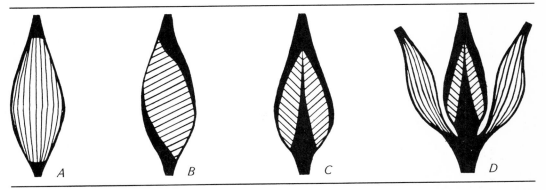

Figure 1-2. Diagrams showing kinds of arrangements of fibers of skeletal muscles. *A,* fusiform. *B,* unipennate. *C,* bipennate. *D,* multipennate. (Douglas.) From Rasch-Burke: *Kinesiology and Applied Anatomy* Fifth Edition, Lea & Febiger, Philadelphia, Pa., 1974. Used by permission.

Muscle Fiber Structure

The muscle cell—the contractile portion of the gross muscle—is surrounded by an extremely thin, semipermeable membrane called the *sarcolemma.* Just beneath the sarcolemma are the cell's *nucleii.* Within the fluid portion of the cell, the *sarcoplasm,* are the *myofibrils.* These myofibrils are the actual contractile units of each fiber, and are columnar structures of alternating light and dark segments. The coloring is due to the relative density of the overlapping protein filaments within each myofibril. Short, thick filaments of the protein *myosin* overlap with long, thin filaments of the protein *actin.* One "section" of these overlapping filaments is called a *sarcomere.*

Other Structural Considerations

There are other structures within each fiber that are related to its function. Tiny organelles, called *mitochondria,* are located between the myofibrils, and are responsible for the oxidative metabolism of the fibers as well as for the production ATP (adenosinetriphosphate). More will be said on this subject later in the chapter. Other

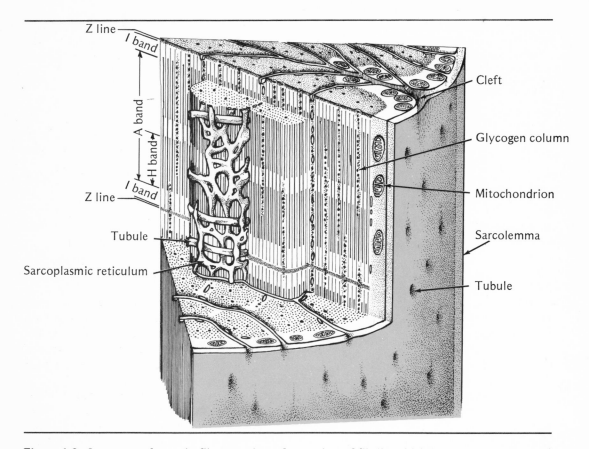

Figure 1-3. Structure of muscle fiber consists of a number of fibrils, which in turn are made up of orderly arrays of thick and thin filaments of protein. A system of transverse tubules opens to the exterior of the fiber. The sarcoplasmic reticulum is a system of tubules that does not open to the exterior. The two systems, which are evidently involved in the flow of calcium ions, meet at a number of junctions called dyads or triads. Mitochondria convert food to energy. The sarcolemma is a membrane surrounding the fiber. From *How Is Muscle Turned On and Off?* by Graham Hoyle. Copyright © 1970 by Scientific American, Inc. All rights reserved.

organelles of interest are the *sarcoplasmic reticulum* and transversely located tubules (called *t-tubules*). The t-tubules open to the exterior of the fiber, and meet with the sarcoplasmic reticulum at strategic locations within the individual myofibrils. The sarcoplasmic reticulum is responsible for the storage and release of calcium ions, and, while the t-tubules are involved in this function also, they also are involved in the even distribution of the nerve impulse which triggers muscular contraction throughout the fiber.

Other, subcellular, structures are of importance also. *Ribosomes* are responsible for protein synthesis, especially during chronic exercise. *Myoglobin,* a red pigment, maintains the proper oxygen concentration within the fibers, allowing the mitochondria to function properly. *Glycogen granules* are located between the myofibrils for easy access, and are the "fuel" for energy production. Finally, various *enzymes* are present, and are collectively associated with the utilization of the glycogen.

Blood Supply to Muscle Fibers

Arteries run from the heart through the spaces between the fasciculii, and branch into smaller *arterioles,* passing through the perimysium into the fasciculii. The arterioles then branch into tiny *capillaries* which service the individual muscle fibers. The exchange of foodstuffs and oxygen for metabolic waste material takes place at this level. The capillaries become *venioles,* and the venioles become *veins,* which return the waste-laden blood to the heart, and eventually to the lungs for elimination of the waste products. It seems somewhat unnecessary to state that the better the blood supply to the individual fibers, the more efficient will be the recovery rate of the exerciser. More will be said on this subject later.

Nerve Supply to Muscle Fibers

The functional unit involved in muscular innervation is the *motor unit*. Each motor unit has associated with it one *neuron* (nerve cell), with its *dendritic tree* and *axon*. The axon is a long, stringlike structure which carries the impulse to the fiber(s) of the motor unit. At the muscle, the axon branches into tiny *twigs,* which run to the individual fibers, and an *end plate* (also referred to as *terminal endings* or as the *myoneural junction*) attaches the twig with the sarcolemma of the fibers (see Figure 1-4).

There may be from one to as many as one hundred separate muscle fibers innervated by a single neuron. Collectively, the neuron and all the muscle cells innervated by it are called a motor unit. An important point to remember is that the muscle fibers of any given motor unit are generally distributed throughout the gross muscle. That is, they are not all located close together. Another important point to remember is that when a motor unit is stimulated, all of the fibers associated with that motor unit contract fully. This is known as the "all-or-none" law of muscular contraction. However, since there are as many as fifty or more stimulations per second, or as few as ten or less, the amount of *tension* developed by the muscle allows for a finely *graded response*. This gradation of response in muscle tension is further facilitated by yet another mechanism called *asynchronous innervation*. Not all motor units are stimulated simultaneously, for if they were, fatigue would set in very rapidly, and all work would necessarily cease. Rather, when the *excitation threshold* of a motor unit is reached, it contracts and then relaxes while other motor units carry on the contraction. Perhaps an example of this mechanism will facilitate understanding. When you lift a fork to your mouth to eat, you initially perceive the weight of the fork to be minimal, and the stimulation is commensurately slight. However, when you perform the same curling movement with a dumbbell, the perception is different, and many more motor units are stimulated due to the greater amount of millivoltage reaching the muscle involved. If the dumbbell were a fake, an embarrassingly large number of motor units would have been stimulated as the weight would literally fly off the floor. This built-in gradation mechanism, then, allows

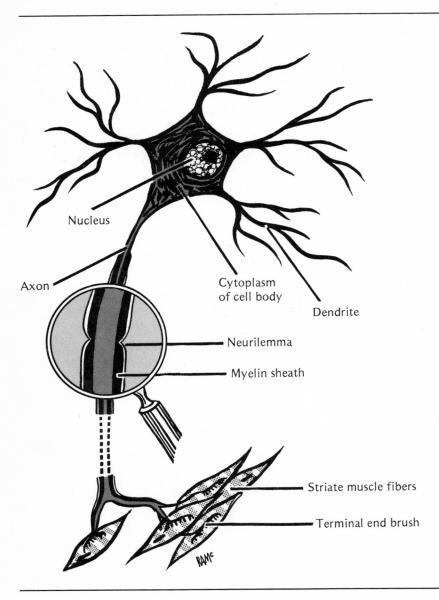

Figure 1-4. A diagrammatic drawing of a neuron. At the top is the cell body and its numerous branchings, the dendrites. They make up the soma of the neuron. The axon, of which there is only one, extends downward. The point at which the axon leaves the soma is the axon hillock. Axons, and sometimes dendrites, may be covered with a myelin sheath, and, outside the nervous system, with a neurilemma. From Morgan and Stellar, *Physiological Psychology*. Copyright © 1950 by McGraw-Hill Book Company. Used by permission.

for both extremely fine movements to occur as well as for allowing muscle fibers a chance to recuperate while others take over.

Generally, the muscles involved in fine movements are comprised of motor units with relatively few muscle fibers, whereas muscles involved in gross movements are comprised of motor units with a great number of muscle fibers. As mentioned earlier, the impulse from the end plate travels down the sarcolemma and throughout the network of t-tubules, allowing for simultaneous stimulation of all of the muscle fiber's myofibrils.

Located between the muscle fibers is an important *proprioceptor* known as the *muscle spindle*. Actually a modified muscle fiber, this mechanism is stimulated when the surrounding muscle fibers are stretched, and the resultant stimulation is sent back to the *alpha motor*

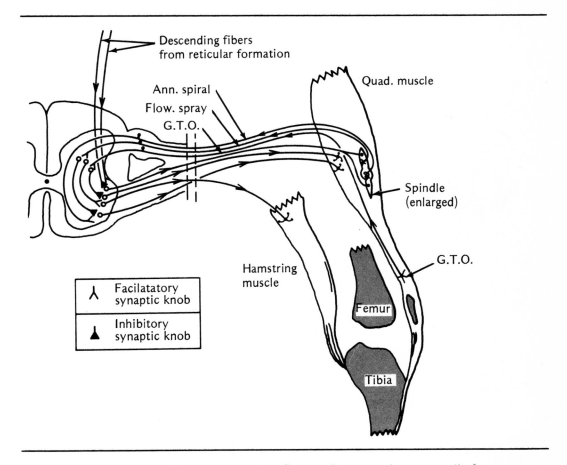

Figure 1-5. The myotatic and inverse myotatic reflexes as "autogenetic governors" of movement at the knee joint. Note that supraspinal influence, both facilitatory and inhibitory is brought to bear on the gamma efferent neuron thus setting the bias of the spindle. From deVries: *Physiology of Exercise* Second Edition. Wm. C. Brown Company Publishers, 1974. Used by permission.

neurons which innervate the same muscle fibers. The appropriate motor units are thereby stimulated, and the muscle contracts in opposition to the original stretch placed on the muscle. This is known as the *stretch reflex,* and has as its most common example the knee-jerk reflex. There are many instances in sport and weight lifting wherein this mechanism may be used to the athlete's advantage. Another point involving this stretch reflex must be discussed before leaving the subject, however. At the same time the stretched muscles are called upon to react to the stretch they have been placed under, other "helping" muscles called *synergists* and *stabilizer* muscles are brought into play also. Their contraction aids the stretched muscles to respond. Also, there is a general inhibition of the stretched muscle's *antagonists*. These are the muscles which are in opposition to the contracting muscle (called the *protagonist* when spoken of in conjunction with the antagonist). For example, when the stretch reflex causes the biceps to contract, the muscles on the back of the arm, the triceps, are simultaneously inhibited from contracting, allowing for facilitated contracture of the bicep. This chain of events is called *reciprocal innervation.*

Working with the muscle spindles is yet another proprioceptor called the *golgi tendon organ*. This mechanism, located in the tendon of the muscle, is stimulated when stretched by a contracting muscle. Its functions are twofold: first, they relay information about the force of contracture to the central nervous system, allowing for just the right amount of force to be applied while lifting an object; secondly, they serve to protect the muscle from damage from excessive tension. This second function is accomplished by inhibiting further contraction of the protagonist, and stimulating a corresponding contracture of the antagonist.

Energetics of Anaerobic and Aerobic Pathways

The energy for muscular contraction is derived from ATP (spoken of earlier in this chapter). As contraction continues, the stores of this organic compound are broken down to produce inorganic compounds and energy (ATP $\longrightarrow$ ADP + P + E). This is the energy used for contraction. However, these ATP stores are quickly depleted, and another organic compound called *phosphocreatine* is broken down so that the energy released in its breakdown can combine with the ADP to resynthesize ATP for additional energy for contraction. This reaction is summarized as follows: CP $\longrightarrow$ C + P + E. Again, however, this process cannot continue, because the CP is also quickly depleted. At this point, glycogen is broken down to yield the energy required to replenish the stores of phosphocreatine so that it can in turn be broken down to resynthesize ATP. As the glycogen is broken down, lactic acid and energy are released. It would now appear that the process is complete; that is, the organic phosphates are continuously resynthesized. The stores of glycogen are also being depleted, however, and lactic acid, a waste product which retards contraction, is accumulating as a result of the glycogen breakdown. The equilibrium of this process, therefore, is not maintained; if it were, muscular contraction could last only about 30 seconds due to the buildup of lactic acid and the depletion of glycogen. Thus far in the process, no oxygen has been used to produce contraction. Therefore, the process to this point is referred to as the *anaerobic* pathway.

Oxygen being introduced into the process allows two more chemical reactions to occur. Oxygen combines with about one-fifth of the built-up lactic acid to produce energy. This energy is used to convert the remaining four-fifths of the lactic acid back into glycogen. The water and carbon dioxide produced in the first reaction are passed off via the circulatory system and expelled by the lungs during normal breathing. The entire chain is summarized in Figure 1-6. It should be clearly understood, however, that both the processes summarized here and in Figure 1-6 are just that—summaries. The reader is directed to any good exercise physiology text for the complete group of reactions which occur. The portion of the reactions summarized which involve the utilization of oxygen is called the *aerobic* pathway. Work can now continue indefinitely, provided that sufficient oxygen is present to interact with the lactic acid.

As work becomes progressively intense, and the circulatory system becomes incapable of supplying sufficient oxygen to oxidize the lactic acid, fatigue sets in. A buildup of less than a few tenths of 1% of the lactic acid concentration in a muscle results in muscular pain and a cessation of contraction. This fatigue is the most commonly experienced type, and is normally accompanied by an *oxygen debt*. Expressing it another way, the amount of oxygen it would take to oxidize the built-up lactic acid is "owed" to the system, and one's "tolerance" for an accumulated debt is generally proportional to his aerobic fitness.

---

1. Organic Phosphate → Inorganic Phosphate + Organic Phosphate + Energy
      ATP   →   P   +   ADP   + Energy
  (Adenosine Tri-   (Phosphate)   (Adenosine Di-
    Phosphate)   Phosphate)

2. Organic Phosphate + Organic Phosphate → Organic Phosphate + Organic Mineral
      CP   +   ADP   →   ATP   +   C
  (Creatine   (Adenosine Di-   (Adenosine Tri-   (Creatine)
    Phosphate)   Phosphate)   Phosphate)

3. Glycogen → Lactic Acid + Energy for resynthesis of CP
       (i.e., for putting 'P' from 1 and 'C' from 2 back together)

4. Organic Mineral + Inorganic Phosphate + Energy → Organic Phosphate
      C   +   P   + Energy →   CP

5. 1/5 Lactic Acid + O_2 → CO_2 + H_2O + Energy for resynthesis of remainder
                                    Lactic Acid

6. 4/5 Lactic Acid + Energy (from 5) + O_2 → Glycogen

Figure 1-6. Summary of anaerobic and aerobic pathways.

Mechanics of Muscular Contraction

In the previously discussed section on muscle cell structure, it was mentioned that muscle fibers consisted of the sarcolemma, nucleii, sarcoplasm, and myofibrils, together with other smaller organelles and subcellular structures. This section deals with the mechanics of myofibrillar contraction.

An electrical impulse arriving at the motor end plate of the fibers causes the release of *acetylcholine* (ACh), a chemical which initiates a disturbance of the permeability of the sarcolemma. This disturbance travels down the sarcolemma and through the t-tubules to release calcium from the sarcoplasmic reticula. Prolonged stimulation causes the vescicles which release the ACh to diminish. However, generally before this can occur, another chemical, *acetylcholinesterase,* destroys the ACh and returns the sarcolemma to its former stability. It is the release of calcium which triggers contraction.

The released calcium binds with a regulatory protein called *troponin,* which is located on the long, thin actin filaments within the myofibrils. This bond causes an interaction between the actin and myosin filaments such that they are forced through a change in conformation. This conformational change involves the production of a "pulling force" between the actin and myosin filaments. The process is reversed upon the destruction of ACh (i.e., upon relaxation).

Prevalent theory in exercise physiology has it that the mechanism involved in the sliding of the actin and myosin filaments across each other to produce muscular contraction is actually similar to tiny "cross bridges" grabbing, releasing, and regrabbing their way across each other (see Figure 1-7). Since the actin filaments are connected to the portion of the sarcomere referred to as the Z line, this pulling action draws the two ends of the sarcomere together. As this process continues, the force exerted by the sliding filaments is transmitted to the connective tissues of the muscle, then to the tendons which act on the bones to which they are attached.

Types of muscular contraction. While the mechanics of muscular contraction are basically the same for all types of contractions, it is necessary to describe their differences. These differences will be vital to a basic understanding of various systems of training, to be discussed in a later chapter.

Isometric contraction of a muscle occurs when the weight being lifted is too heavy to move (e.g., pushing against a brick wall or pulling at a weight which is too heavy to budge). In this instance, cross bridging occurs, but not to the extent that movement is caused, or, rather, not to the extent that a shortening of the muscle occurs.

Isotonic contraction, on the other hand, does involve an actual shortening of the muscle. This process is clearly illustrated during the "curling" of a weight held in the hand. You will notice the biceps bulge at the middle while the weight is being lifted. This bulge is the result of the sarcomeres being drawn toward one another during the cross-bridging process. The shortening of the muscle during isotonic contraction is referred to as *concentric* contraction, because of the acted-upon limb's movement toward the contracting muscle. When the same weight used in the example above is lowered, another form of isotonic contraction is involved—*eccentric* contraction. In eccentric contraction, the cross bridges apparently are raked across each other in an effort to shorten, but the intensity, or frequency, of innervation is not great enough to allow this to happen. This "raking" is similar to pulling two toothbrushes across one another, and it results in a high amount of friction. This concept will be referred to again later in the text. It has been found that concentric contraction of a muscle involves considerably more motor units than does eccentric contraction, a fact which

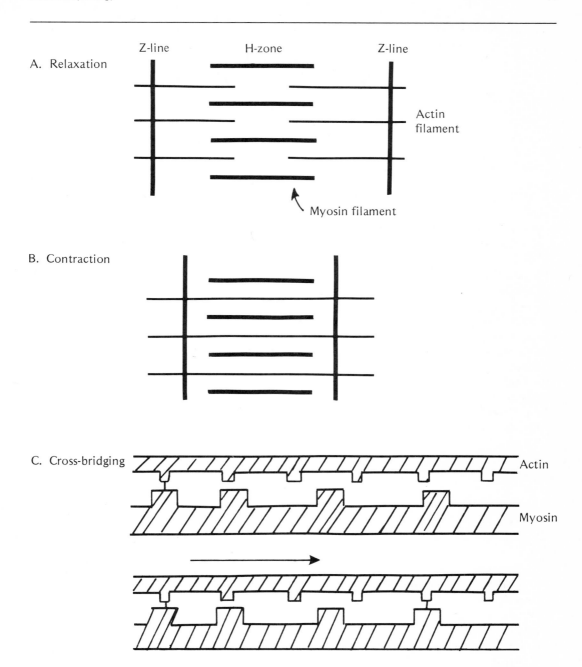

Figure 1-7. Representation of the "cross-bridging" theory of contraction (labelled).

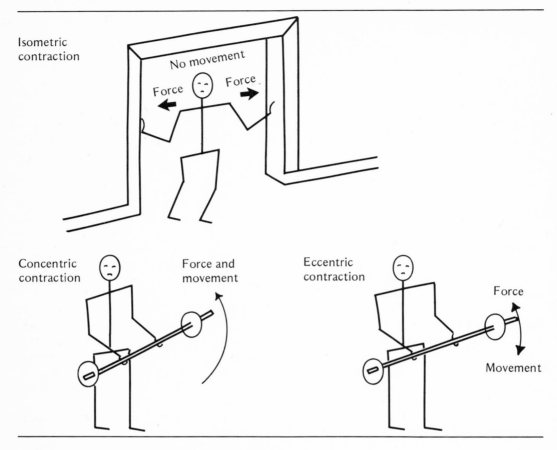

Figure 1-8. Diagram of different types of contraction (labelled).

explains the relatively greater energy expenditure during concentric work. However, this phenomenon applies only if the same amount of weight are involved in both forms of contraction. Far greater amounts of weight can be lowered in an eccentric movement, for example, than can be lifted during a concentric movement. This has prompted some weight trainers to use a system of training involving the use of eccentric contracture. The term used to describe this method of training has been *negative resistance* training, to which further reference will be made later in the text.

Types of Muscle Fiber

The last time you dined on chicken, did you prefer the dark meat or did you dig in to the white portion? Have you ever wondered why such differentiation of muscle tissue occurs? Chickens are ground birds, so their wing muscles (the breast) are adapted to short, power flights only, and their legs are correspondingly adapted to bearing their weight. The same type of differentiation of muscle tissue is present in man, although species-related considerations must be accounted for.

Red muscle fiber, or, *slow-twitch* fiber, has greater oxidative capacity than does white muscle fiber, or, *fast-twitch*. That is, slow-twitch fibers have a greater endurance capacity. The endurance of a muscle is closely related to the size and number of mitochondria, the extent of capillarization around the fibers, the concentration of glycogen stores, and the concentration of myoglobin. The myoglobin is responsible for the red coloration of slow-twitch muscle fibers. These factors enable the muscle to produce energy for contraction over a long period of time since anaerobic and aerobic pathways are considerably enhanced by the presence of these factors.

The speed and tension of muscular contraction, however, are dependent on properties which differ from those involved in muscular endurance. The speed at which a muscle contracts is closely related to the rate at which ATP can be utilized; and this ability is related to the presence of related enzymes and the extensiveness of the sarcoplasmic reticulum network. The amount of tension produced by a muscle (that is, the strength of the muscle's contraction) is also closely related to enzyme activity, but other less apparent factors are more important. The amount of myofibrillar protein per cross-sectional area is important, for example. So, too, is the number of muscle fibers in the muscle as well as the number of fibers in each motor unit.

Thus, a three-way classification system has emerged, involving the speed, tension, and endurance of muscle fibers. With regard to speed, white muscle fibers appear to be best suited, but they vary considerably, however, in their endurance capacity. A muscle fiber may be fast-twitch, and have high- or low-oxidative capacity, or it may be slow-twitch. Generally, slow-twitch fibers vary less than fast-twitch in their oxidative capacity—all are generally fatigue resistant. The tension capacity of a muscle is closely related to the speed of contraction. Thus, fast-twitch fibers are generally also the strongest.

Another point should be made regarding the speed capacity of slow- and fast-twitch fibers. There is some speculation that the relatively thicker nerves servicing the fast-twitch fibers are responsible for their greater shortening speed. This point tends to corroborate what experience has shown the majority of weight trainers—that selection of specific types of exercises performed at specific speeds, intensities and durations have selective effects on the different muscle fiber types. One can train specifically for endurance, speed and/or strength. More will be said on this principle of specificity later.

While certain types of exercise can cause changes in concentrations of various factors within a muscle fiber (e.g., fast-twitch fibers that had a low-oxidative capacity can become fast-twitch with a higher oxidative capacity), the ratio of fast-twitch and slow-twitch fibers is genetically determined, and cannot be changed through training. Biopsies performed on champion sprinters and long-distance swimmers confirm the fact that this inherited ratio predetermines an athlete's capacity to achieve in these activities. The sprinter was born with a preponderance of fast-twitch fibers, while the long-distance swimmer inherited a preponderance of the red, slow-twitch fibers that are suited to endurance activity. Many countries are now engaged in preselection of athletes for certain sports, basically through reference to these considerations. While such preselection techniques have obvious advantages, it seems that in our society, with strong pressures to preserve such basic human rights as freedom of choice, such practices are, at best, in the distant future.

Basic Principles of Training

2

Chapter 1 dealt with the structural and functional mechanisms of muscular contraction. The basic principles described therein are the basis for selecting and performing exercise regimen. One cannot expect to increase a muscle's power, for example, by performing exercises which isolate red fibers. White fibers are most important in power movements, and red are called upon primarily in endurance efforts. Thus, a basic group of principles emerges which will aid the exerciser in achieving personal fitness objectives in an efficient and maximized manner.

Basic Principles of Weight Training

Probably the most basic principle of exercise is that the body grows in efficiency and size with exercise, and deteriorates with disuse. This is referred to as the *law of use and disuse*. This law can be clearly seen by observing the circumference of a limb before and after it has been placed in a cast for several weeks. The limb's musculature undergoes severe *atrophy,* and the joints become relatively immobile. Mobility is returned only after weeks of use, and the muscles also return to their previous size after a similar period of time and use. Muscles adapt to the demands placed upon them in highly specific ways. That is, muscles will adapt to endurance requirements through endurance training, and will not, during that process, undergo significant changes in other areas such as speed or strength. This phenomenon is referred to as the *SAID principle* (Specific Adaptation to Imposed Demands).

Adaptation generally involves another dimension also—that of overcompensation. Callus builds up in the hands as an adaptation to friction, muscle fibrils which are splintered during heavy exercise grow in both size and number, and lacerated tissue develops new "scar" tissue in greater amounts than the original tissue. These are examples of a specific class of adaptation responses referred to as the *law of overcompensation*.

Related to these basic principles is the notion that adaptation and overcompensation can

15

occur only if the particular structure is taxed beyond that level which it normally is accustomed to. Adaptation must be forced to occur. By progressively increasing the stress placed on the muscles, one forces the muscles to adapt. This is referred to as the *overload principle.*

Since many human forms of movement require the use of many different muscles, it seems that only the weaker muscles involved in the movement are being taxed maximally, the stronger ones bearing the stresses of the movement with ease. These larger or stronger muscles will not adapt to great stress unless great stress is placed upon them. Consequently, there must be some means of isolating them so as to alleviate the problem of smaller, weaker muscles limiting the amount of stress that can be placed on them. In weight training, this need is accounted for by the array of exercises and specialized apparatuses used. The *isolation principle* is the key to selecting the appropriate exercise, while the SAID and overload principles are the keys to how that exercise should be performed.

With the preceding principles in mind, we can now progress to a discussion of the specific factors involved in training, and basic methods of achieving desired outcomes.

Factors Involved in Muscular Strength

Generally, the strength of contraction of a single muscle fiber is related to the ability of the contractile elements to contract, producing tension. As was discussed earlier, fast-twitch muscle fibers are generally more capable of producing higher tension than are red, slow-twitch fibers, presumably due to more efficient enzyme activity and nerve fiber properties. It is not clear as to whether there is a direct causal relationship between strength and fiber hypertrophy; nor is it clear whether hypertrophy of individual fibers is due to increased size and numbers of myofibrils or to an increase in the amount of sarcoplasm, or both. It is, however, a purely theoretical concept at this level. What is really important is the strength of the entire muscle and the amount of force that can be produced at the ends of the bony levers.

Gross muscular strength is related to (1) the arrangement of muscle fibers (i.e., fusiform or penniform), (2) the number of motor units being stimulated simultaneously, (3) the preponderance of white versus red fibers, and (4) an innominate factor, involving what may be considered social and psychological motivation and the ability of the exerciser to concentrate on the specific muscle being contracted. In any event, the fourth factor probably can be reduced to the fact that more motor units are recruited in the effort.

The amount of force that can be produced at the ends of the bony levers, however, involves additional factors. Coordinating the actions of all the muscles involved in the movement, for example, will result in greater force application. This coordinated effort involves the *prime movers,* the helping *synergists,* and the *stabilizers.* Prime movers are those muscles whose fibers are arranged such that their contraction most aids the movement, and synergistic muscles are those whose fibers help, but only minimally, due to their nonadvantageous angle of pull. Stabilizer muscles contract isometrically to render other body parts immovable during the desired movement, and are generally located nearer the origin of the prime movers.

The efficiency of the lever system involved is of paramount importance. An example of such leverage is illustrated in Figure 2-1. Notice that if the force arm (distance between mus-

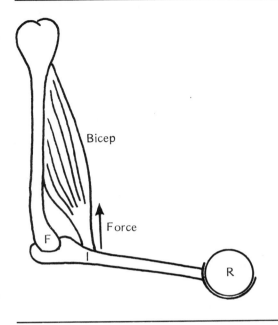

F = Fulcrum
I = Muscle's insertion
R = Resistance (16 pound shot)
force arm = FI (2 inches)
resistance arm = RF (14 inches)

force X FI = R X RF

force X 2 = 16 X 14

force X 2 = 224

force = 112 pounds

If F I were 3 inches, however,

force X 3 = 224

force = 74.67 pounds

Thus, less force is needed to lift the same weight when the insertion point is located farther down the forearm.

Figure 2-1. The arm acting as a third class lever, and formula for determining the amount of force applied.

cle's insertion and the axis) is lengthened, the resultant force will be greater. This general principle holds true for most of the lever systems in the body, as only a few of them are other than third-class levers. Needless to say, the length of any given force arm is an inherited trait. One can readily see the advantage an athlete with good leverage would have over one who didn't. Far more muscular force is needed by athletes lacking efficient leverage in order to lift the same amount of weight.

With the preceding knowledge regarding the source(s) of muscular strength, it should become quite clear that, in most activities, strength alone is of little value. Explosive strength, on the other hand, is essential. *Power* is the rate of doing work, while strength is merely the amount of force which a muscle is able to produce. Thus, power can be thought of as being resultant of two factors, speed, which increases the rate at which force can be applied, and strength, which produces the force. One has, therefore, three methods at his disposal by which to increase power: (1) increase his strength, (2) increase his speed, or (3) increase both. While speed can be improved, the amount of improvement will be minimal. Generally, speed increments are a result of learning to coordinate efforts of muscles involved, and learning to achieve maximal recruitment of appropriate fibers. Thus, since such learning normally occurs rapidly, noticeable gains in speed are made, after which gains become minimal. Strength, on the other hand, can be increased markedly and over a long period of time—most athletes have not begun to realize their strength potential.

Methods of Strength Development

The amount of *tension* produced by a muscle is the key to significant strength increases. Research has indicated that, for explosive strength to increase, loads of greater than two-thirds of one's maximal limit must be used, and 80%-90% of one's maximum being generally recommended. Since the fuel for such activity is the organic phosphates ATP and CP, which are depleted very rapidly during explosive movements, the *duration* and *frequency* of the exercise must be such that these energy substrate are resynthesized. Should contractions continue beyond about ten seconds, aerobic mechanisms take over, and the amount of tension developed by the muscle generally falls below the critical two-thirds limit. Consequently, four to six repetitions (completed in less than ten seconds) are recommended. There should be a brief rest between sets to allow resynthesis of ATP and CP to occur. About 3-6 sets of 4-6 repetitions should be performed, again with near-maximum weight. Each repetition should be performed explosively, to accomodate the learning factor.

Upon repeated depletion of energy substrate, overcompensation takes place. That is, stores of ATP and CP become more abundant. This allows one to continue contraction for a longer period, perhaps, but is not related to increased muscular strength. This is what is called *strength endurance,* not to be confused with muscular or cardiovascular endurance. Again, strength increases are due to the learning factor and to the increased efficiency, or the *quality,* of the myofibrillar elements in producing tension.

It should be pointed out that strength training is highly specific. Only the motor units involved will benefit from exercise, and it is maximum effort per repetition which stimulates

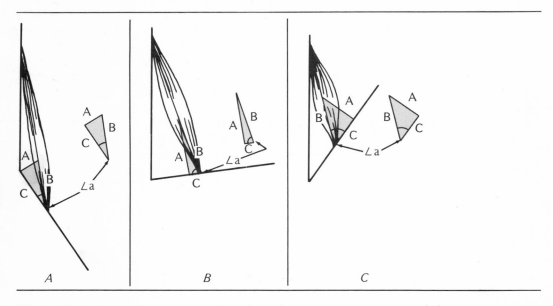

Figure 2-2. Effect of the angle of pull of a muscle upon the external force (A) provided for equal amounts of internal muscular force (B). Side (C) in each case represents wasted internal force. From deVries: *Physiology of Exercise* Second Edition. Wm. C. Brown Company Publishers, 1974. Used by permission.

other, previously unused, motor units. Furthermore, such training will not improve the tension capacity of other muscles—only those involved in the overload process will benefit significantly. During isotonic contractions of the type mentioned above, only a very small portion of the total movement will be overloaded if the degree of effort remains constant over the entire movement. This is true because the angle of the muscle's insertion into the bony lever determines how much weight can be lifted. For example, the elbow joint is stronger at 90° than it is at 120° or 60° of flexion. Consequently, the muscle is being overloaded only during the portion of the movement wherein the muscle is weakest. To circumvent this problem, one must attempt to maximally contract the biceps throughout the full range of movement, and must, correspondingly, accelerate the movement to such a degree that the ballistic, or momentum, factor is minimized. What the exerciser must strive to do, therefore, is to recruit as large a number of motor units as possible at every angle throughout the movement, thus allowing for efficient overload at every angle.

Factors Involved in Muscular Hypertrophy

The most noticeable effect of weight training is that muscles grow larger with time. This effect is called *hypertrophy,* and is generally due to the overcompensation principle. Again, as in strength development, muscles grow by applying overload, and only those fibers directly stimulated will hypertrophy. It is probable that all elements of the muscle are increased through hypertrophy training. The myofibrils increase in size and number, the connective tissues become thicker, sarcoplasmic content is increased, and increased numbers of capillaries are caused to appear. Thus, for maximal hypertrophy, variation in exercise methods is important, since many of the muscle's elements are increased in size, number, quantity and/or function differentially.

The site of myofibrillar hypertrophy may reside in the nervous system. As mentioned earlier (Chapter 1), the nerves which service white, fast-twitch fibers are thicker than those which service the red, slow-twitch fibers. This anatomical difference, it is believed, accounts for the fast- versus slow-twitch properties of the respective fibers. This fact also tends to explain why white fiber myofibrils have the capacity for greater hypertrophy than do the red fibers myofibrils.

On the other hand, red fibers, rich in myoglobin, mitochondria, and capillaries, are more suited to aerobic work than are the white fibers. There are some white fibers, however, which possess high-oxidative capacity similar to the red fibers. While they are fast-twitch, they also are fatigue-resistant. By taxing their fatigue resistance via overload endurance training, these fibers respond by becoming more resistant to fatigue through developing greater amounts of myoglobin and capillaries.

Since the tension produced by the myofibrils causes a pull at all of the surrounding connective tissues and the muscle's tendons, a thickening of the connective tissue and tendons occurs so as to compensate for the increased tension placed on them. Again we see the principle of overcompensation operating. Generally, forceful, fast contractions will cause this thickening as well as the increased hypertrophy of the myofibrillar elements, while slow, submaximal, continuous contractions will cause increases in oxygen demands of the red fibers, thereby causing increases in capillaries, myoglobin, mitochondria, and enzyme concentrations.

Methods of Hypertrophy Development

As pointed out earlier, variation of method is a key concept in training for hypertrophy. The greatest amount of muscular hypertrophy stems from the overcompensation effect of increased size and number of myofibrillar elements within the muscle fiber. High-speed work with a load of 60% of one's maximum for about 15 repetitions and 4-6 sets will yield this effect, but the strength and muscular endurance benefits will be minimal. For strength to increase along with increases in hypertrophy, loads of 80% or greater must be used. This system involves doing high-speed movements for about 6-8 repetitions for a similar number of sets. Again, recall that tension is the key to strength development; it is assumed that far more weight can be handled if the number of repetitions performed is low. At the other end of the spectrum, performing an exercise for 30 or more repetitions with extremely light weights (less than 40%), and maintaining a slow, continuous cadence, is more suited to developing the red fibers' elements—the mitochondria, capillaries, myoglobin, and enzymes. Additionally, this type of training will tend to convert many of the white, fast-twitch fibers to the point where their oxidative capacity is increased. Far less hypertrophy occurs in such a system than in ones involving strictly fast-twitch fibers. In fact, should one regress in load to below 40%, and maintain or increase the number of repetitions performed, an actual decrease in both size and strength is generally noted.

Many lifters interested in hypertrophy (or body-building, as it is commonly called) rely on a system of training called *forced repetition* training. Here, the lifter performs his exercise to fatigue, and then, by sheer willpower or concentration, forces his muscles to repond by performing two or more additional repetitions. Such a system seems at odds with the principle of avoiding fatigue (mentioned under strength development), since the critical percentage of maximum would not be achieved. However, the theory is that by forcing out additional repetitions, one calls upon as yet unused motor units to respond, thereby lowering their threshold of excitation so that they can be called upon with greater ease later. As this process continues, recruitment of such unused fibers becomes more and more difficult. The cliche that one must "train through pain in order to gain" is a widespread belief in the world of body-building, and such a system has produced the greatest physique artists in history. Notwithstanding this notion's popularity, however, for *complete* development to occur, variations in the forced repetitions system of the type already mentioned are recommended. In other words, forced repetitions can be done while performing the 40%, 60%, or 80% systems—there need not be any disagreement on this point.

Inasmuch as hypertrophy training requires a rather diversified program, involving elements from both strength and endurance training as well as some elements unique to itself, it is the system most recommended for the general fitness enthusiast. Moderate gains in both strength and muscular and strength endurance components can be realized along with a more appealing physique. Body-building, as an art and sport, has far surpassed weight lifting in popularity in this country, and the various benefits which can be derived are probably at the root of this popularity. For overall fitness, however, one must consider the cardiovascular and cardiorespiratory systems as well. More will be said on the matter of overall physical fitness later in the text.

Factors Involved in Muscular Endurance

The adaptive changes which take place as a result of endurance training overlap only minimally with those occurring during strength and hypertrophy training. Very little size and strength increase takes place in such training, as the adaptations occur largely under the umbrella of the aerobic pathway. It is entirely possible for muscular endurance to increase substantially as a result of strength and hypertrophy training, but far more efficient and complete muscular endurance development can be obtained through calling upon the aerobic pathway. That is, by overloading the muscles so that their need for oxygen is increased, adaptation of the mechanisms involved in the oxidative process are increased in size, numbers and/or function.

Repeated, submaximal contractions cause a reddening of some of the white fibers are a result of increased myoglobin concentrations, and also cause the red fibers to become redder. Recall that the myoglobin's function was to maintain a proper oxygen concentration in the fibers. However, for this to be possible, there must be more oxygen. Adaptive increases occur, therefore, in the size and numbers of mitochondria, which are responsible for the oxidative metabolism of the muscle as well as the synthesis of ATP. Also, an adaptive buildup of capillaries surrounding the fiber occurs. New capillaries are thought to be formed as a result of the continued contraction; it is also possible that other, previously dormant, capillaries are opened through the same process. The muscle's glycogen stores are also elevated. Additionally, changes occur within the nervous system which are designed to allow greater repetition of, or greater length of, muscular contraction. In any case, noted gains in strength or size as a result of endurance training are visible only initially (probably as a result of reversing some of the effects of disuse), and are minimal at that. They do not continue to increase beyond the first two or three weeks of training.

Methods of Muscular Endurance Development

While the keys to strength training and hypertrophy training are tension and variation, respectively, the key to muscular endurance training is oxygen utilization and transport. For these factors to become maximized, both the frequency and duration of the exercise must be high. The speed at which each repetition is to be performed should coincide, as nearly as possible, with the activity for which muscular endurance is sought, while the number of repetitions should not exceed 40 or 50 (before the intensity of one's effort begins to decline). For example, a bicyclist, concerned about his leg muscles' capacity to continue sustained and repeated contractions during an all-out sprint race, or a swimmer, wishing to achieve local muscular endurance in his shoulder muscles for a 100-meter butterfly event, would, as closely as possible, approximate the speed at which their respective activities are performed during the weight training sessions. Further, in order to derive maximal benefit in this regard, sufficient weight would be used such that around 40 or 50 repetitions could be performed at that speed. Dipping below the required speed would be analogous to slowing down a required speed in their respective athletic events. By training in this manner, overcompensation is forced on the muscles involved in the general capacity of that muscle to utilize oxygen, as well as in the circulatory system's capacity to deliver greater amounts of oxygen.

Figure 2-3. The different athletic endeavors depicted here require different physical attributes. The wise coach or athlete should identify the components of fitness most essential in his/her sport, and select the most appropriate avenue to acquire them. One of the important points of this text is to point out the importance of adhering to the basic principles of conditioning, whatever the desired outcome or avenue chosen to achieve it.

A. These swimmers are competing in the butterfly event. The short distance covered in this event necessitates concentrating on both power as well as local muscular endurance, while other events covering greater distances would require cardiovascular endurance primarily.

B. This high jumper must possess exceptional leg power to propel his body upwards. Other muscles, acting as synergists (or, helpers) must be powerful also, including lower back and arm elevator muscles. The so-called "Fosbury Flop" technique requires exceptional coordination as well.

C. Aside from the high degree of coordination required to put the shot, this woman athlete must possess explosive power in all body segments, in order that the sum of all muscular forces generated while crossing the circle are transferred maximally to the shot. Weight training techniques for women are identical to those engaged in by male athletes. The outburst of record-breaking performances in recent years by women athletes can be traced to the acceptance of weight training as an essential part of their training regimen.

D. This Olympic-style weightlifter has just consumated a successful 300-pound press (a lift no longer contested in international competition). Olympic weightlifters must possess exceptional explosive power, strength and strength endurance. Note the extent of muscular hypertrophy in comparison to that of the high jumper, requiring only leg power.

E. Cross-country running requires cardiovascular and cardiorespiratory endurance. The slim physique of the runner bespeaks the importance of red (slow-twitch) muscle fiber, while the weightlifter depicted here requires primarily white (fast-twitch) muscle fiber.

F. Crew members (coxswain excluded) are generally taller than average, and possess great amounts of local muscular endurance in the legs, lower back, shoulders and biceps. The high number of repetitions necessitates that this attribute be worked on in training. Weight training is, because of the more efficient overload involved, more suited to developing this quality than simply rowing.

G. Here, the gymnast is executing an "L" iron cross, a superior strength move in still rings competition. The gymnast must possess tremendous strength in the muscles of the shoulder girdle as well as in the abdominal region. A case can be made for the necessity for the athlete to possess strength endurance as well, since the position must be held for a sustained period of time.

While little overlap is involved in mechanisms or methods employed in strength versus muscular endurance training, there is some evidence that the stronger a person is, the more likely that his muscular endurance will be high also. This statement makes reference to the difference between *absolute* endurance and *relative* endurance. If two people, one weak and the other strong, held a weight (say, 25 pounds) at arms' length, the stronger of the two would probably be capable of doing so for a longer period than the weaker. This is referred to as absolute endurance. In this case, strength and endurance are correlated highly. However, if each of the two were asked to perform the same exercise with a given percentage of their maximum capacity, no such correlation exists, and we speak of each person's relative endurance. Notwithstanding this difference in terminology, from a purely practical point of view it would be to one's advantage to be strong, since in the real world of performance, absolute rather than relative differences are generally applied. While the stronger

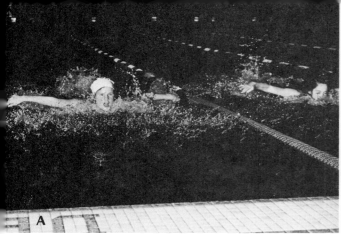

A

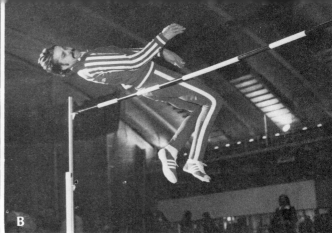

B

Courtesy of James L. Shaffer

Courtesy of University of Wisconsin

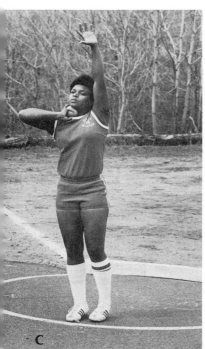

C

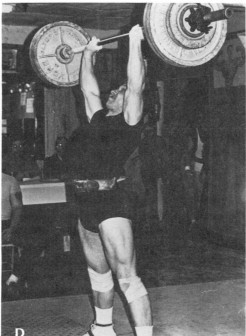

D

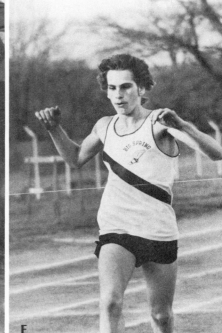

E

Courtesy of Southern Connecticut State College

Courtesy of Strix Pix

Courtesy of Lynn D. Howell

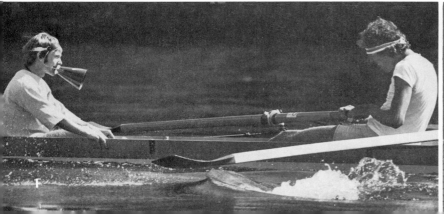

F

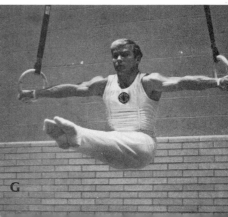

G

person would probably have more abundant stores of the high energy substrates ATP and creatine phosphate, the more likely explanation of this phenomenon is that the protein troponin, which, as we saw earlier, is connected to the actin filaments for interaction with the calcium ions during contraction, becomes inactive as a result of increased acidity within the muscle fiber, thereby causing a decrement in that muscle's contractility. This increased acidity would not occur as quickly in the trained individual.

Factors Involved in Athletic Ability

The factors involved in athletic ability are many, and range in nature from the physiological to the psychological and sociological. Further, it seems necessary to point out that an athlete engaged in one sport may require completely different attributes than athletes in another sport, or even in the same sport but playing a different position. The following discussion, therefore, will be general; it is left up to the reader to ferret out those factors which he or she requires. Further, the list of factors discussed in this section by no means exhausts those which may be essential in sport; nor is it endemic to athletes. The general fitness enthusiast may find it helpful as well.

Before we proceed, however, there are some basic principles which should be considered by the athlete, regardless of the sport or activity engaged in. First, training regimen will vary during preseason, in-season, and off-season periods. Preseason training should be structured such that preparation for competition is the goal. Those attributes most directly involved in successful participation should be honed to a fine edge during this period. The length of the preseason training period should be generally low, not exceeding 6-8 weeks. This is true because high-intensity training routines should be predominant; and should training in this manner continue longer, staleness or overtraining may result. High-intensity training generally involves applying greater and greater overload to the organism. For example, the sprint swimmer may reduce laps and increase speed per lap, the weight lifter may decrease repetitions and increase the amount lifted per repetition, or the long-distance runner may decrease the rest between intervals.

In-season training should be primarily concerned with maintenance of the factors trained for in the preseason and off-season. Power, for example, can be maintained by training only once or twice per week, performing maximal or near-maximal lifts. Should all training cease during the competition season, many of the hard-won gains will become diminished due to the law of use and disuse. Generally, one's actual activity does not offer sufficient overload to allow for maintenance of vital factors. Should the athlete continue to train 3-6 times weekly, on the other hand, the combined effect of training and competing may cause overtraining. Once or twice weekly is sufficient.

Off-season training regimen should be as broad as possible, incorporating all those factors deemed essential to adequate performance, and specifically those factors which appeared lacking during the competition season. A good coach may observe that his players (or individual players) lacked flexibility while performing their respective activities. He would, in the off-season training period, incorporate exercises specifically designed to increase flexibility.

Throughout all seasons, skill requirements are generally attended to, although as stated previously, frequency, duration, and intensity of effort must be considered to alleviate staleness and overtraining. The preceding guidelines governing preseason, in-season, and off-season training regimen are not limited to weight training. They appear to be justifiable and appropriate in cases where little or no weight training is employed as well. Given the scope of this text, however, consideration is given only to weight-training regimen.

All athletes must consider their specific activity's requirements. Having isolated them, the SAID, overload, and isolation principles must be applied in selecting and performing the appropriate exercises. The athlete requiring great power would be making a sad mistake to train for purely strength or local muscular endurance. Gains come slowly, and much time can be saved by prudent and judicious applications of these principles. Correspondingly, the same athlete must consider those muscles involved in his event. For a sprinter to train upper body muscles exclusively, without training for leg power, would be ludicrous.

Power. While this factor has already been discussed in a preceding section, there are certain aspects which relate to athletics that should be pointed out. As noted, speed and strength of contraction are the components of power. Some athletes (e.g., a quarterback) should accentuate the speed factor, while others (e.g., the lineman) should train more specifically for the strength component. Such differential treatment of power exercises simply involves reductions or increases in the load such that the speed at which the respective athlete's activities are performed are closely approximated.

Hypertrophy. While athletes may not be interested in attaining a physique similar to a "Mr. America," it is true that many sports require huge musculature for reasons of efficiency in performance. More importantly, however, strength and power are attained more easily once the appropriate amount of hypertrophy is attained. Gymnasts and wrestlers, together with many other athletes, place a premium on being light. However, they should nonetheless be muscular, keeping their body fat content to a minimum. Needless to say, nutrition plays an important role in such considerations, but nutrition alone cannot supply needed muscle tissue—only training can do that.

Speed. There still exists the myth that weight training (especially weight training for hypertrophy) is detrimental to athletic ability because speed and flexibility is impaired. As was discussed earlier in this chapter, speed can actually be facilitated through weight training, and increased muscular size may, in fact, add to that muscle's capacity to respond at maximum speeds. While somewhat unscientific, the analogy that the bigger the engine is, the more powerful it can be, applies.

Flexibility. Flexibility is defined as the ability of a joint to flex and extend through its full intended range of movement. Factors which may limit flexibility are many. Coaches speak of an athlete being "loose" or "tight" during performance. It has been suggested that tightness results from resistance of antagonistic muscles and their connective tissues. However, such a situation need not have been the result of weight training since, if anything, weight training would have "taught" the antagonists to relax during contraction of protagonists. This concept hinges on neuromuscular coordination, and repeated practice of a movement generally facilitates its development. In the case of weight training, there must be a two-way street in this process, however. In attempting to contract the tricep, which is the antagonist of the bicep, the same faciliatory response must have been practiced. Thus, in order to maintain flexibility in the joints acted upon by these muscles, both protagonists and antagonists must be exercised.

Impaired flexibility resulting from injury or genetic factors, or even from shortened muscles such as may occur from faulty posture or restricted movement can be improved through weight training. By strengthening the muscle which is antagonistic to the shortened (or injured) muscle, not only is the neuromuscular coordination improved, but the added pull by the strengthened muscle tends to offset the inordinate pull of the other.

Again, however, as in power, flexibility requirements may differ among different types of athletes. In fact, improved flexibility may be actually detrimental in some sports. The wise coach or athlete should identify his or her specific requirements in all factors influencing performance.

While weight training may be designed to facilitate flexibility, the standard method of stretching must be considered as the most efficient method. Here, the muscle is stretched so that the stretch reflex (see Chapter 1) is bypassed via sustained pull, and the golgi tendon organ is stimulated to cause a general inhibition of contracture of the muscle under stretch. To facilitate this series of events, extreme concentration on relaxing the stretched muscle seems to be helpful as well.

Skill. As was discussed, repetition of movements tends to increase both the precision as well as the efficiency of movement. Unnecessary contractures of antagonistic muscles tend to be decreased, and the desired movements become more automatic. Similarly, the amounts of energy substrate are significantly reduced due to the increased efficiency, thereby making the movements' costs, in terms of endurance, minimal. Since weight training tends to heighten the sensory stimulation (via the muscle spindles and golgi tendon organs) and to facilitate stimulation of appropriate motor units, skill, in the sense of the word described above, will be enhanced. It should be pointed out, however, that weight-training regimen designed for skill enhancement should be such that each exercise conforms exactly to the movements of the actual skill, both in pattern as well as speed. Only the amount of resistance should be increased. If the amount of weight is such that the speed of movement necessarily falls short of that at which the skill is normally performed, one should at least strive to keep the intensity of effort from faltering to the point of fatigue. Fatigue causes (often imperceptible) changes in the movement patterns being exercised, thereby rendering the athlete's efforts wasted or potentially detrimental.

Agility. Agility is the ability to exert a series of power vents (i.e., to change direction rapidly). As such, the same considerations as were discussed under speed and power should be adhered to. Another dimension which comes to bear in athletic performance of agility movements, however, is that of balance. Balance relates specifically to the location of one's center of gravity during stationary (static) or moving (dynamic) skills performances. Other than noting that a stronger, more powerful person can maintain required positions during static or dynamic skills, a detailed discussion of this attribute is beyond the scope of this text.

Endurance. Most coaches, and certainly most laymen, speak of endurance without regard for the differential mechanisms underlying it. Thus far in this text, differences between strength endurance and local muscular endurance were discussed, as were the methods of achieving them. Much current controversy exists as to whether weight training can contribute significantly to these types of endurance. While the mechanisms and methods of achieving CV and CR endurance are beyond the scope of this text (the reader is referred to any good exercise physiology text for in-depth coverage), the following guidelines should be helpful nonetheless.

As in local muscular endurance, which involves primarily aerobic capacity, CR and CV endurance is involved in oxygen transport and utilization. There are other parameters which come into play, however. *Maximum volume of oxygen uptake* (called max VO_2 uptake), or, the amount of oxygen consumption in the muscles, is due to (1) cardiac output, and (2) increased extraction of the oxygen from the blood at the muscles. Cardiac output generally depends on two not necessarily coincident factors, *heart rate,* (beats per minute) and *stroke volume* (amount of blood pumped out of the heart on each beat). Both appear to be somewhat related to the extraction factor (i.e., the extent of capillarization around the fibers). However, maximal stroke volume can be increased without a commensurate change in heart rate, and vice versa, simply because the trained heart, which can hypertrophy like any other trained muscle, becomes stronger, thereby more capable of pumping greater volumes of blood with each beat during strenuous exercise.

An increase in plasma volume is also noted after training. This effect serves to decrease blood viscosity, making it easier to flow through the tiny capillaries, thereby decreasing the cardiac work required. Hemoglobin (red, oxygen-carrying blood cells) count appears to be related to body size rather than to training effects, and increases in red blood cell count have not been conclusively linked with greater VO_2 uptake capacity. Many athletes have, of late, used a method of *blood doping* to achieve greater endurance, a practice not entirely condoned nor proven efficacious. This practice involves the extraction of blood from the athlete weeks before a meet, and reinjecting it into his system just before the meet in the hopes that the increased hemoglobin count would give him greater endurance.

While some training effect in respiratory efficiency is noted as a result of training, this effect appears to be limited to more efficient breathing patterns. This increased ventilation efficiency allows one to take in less air with heavy training, since the deeper breathing pattern more effectively ventilates the alveoli of the lungs (the tiny air sacs). Vital capacity (the amount of air one can breathe in), and the diffusing capacity of the lungs are thought to be unchanged as a result of training, and are more probably due to heredity.

Thus, it is clear that the locus for increased endurance resides primarily in the heart and muscles. Generally, nonrestrictive activities such as running will increase cardiac function more efficiently than will other, more restrictive exercises such as cycling or weight training. This is due to the fact that tension placed on the muscles restricts blood flow through the capillaries, thereby obviating the necessity of the heart to increase its stroke volume. In other words, recent evidence has been presented that indicates heart rate alone is not a sufficient situation to induce cardiac adaptation—stroke volume must be involved also.

Some weight-training methods are designed to maintain heart rates at or above 150 beats per minute, in the expectation that such a training regimen will yield both CV as well as muscular benefits. There is some evidence that this is possible, in spite of a few conflicting reports. These training regimen, including *circuit training* and *interval training,* will be presented in the next chapter.

Notes on Legends, Stereotypes and Old Wives' Tales

Over the years, many beliefs concerning weight lifting, weight lifters, and what can and cannot be accomplished have been handed down not unlike fables and myths are. While many of these beliefs are based on fact, they are generally muddled to the extent that general comprehension of reality is impossible. Many, too, are based on personal experiences which have little to offer by way of objectivity. Many of these beliefs are presented in this section, with the ultimate goal of dispelling those which have no basis in fact, and shedding light on those which do.

Will weight training cause muscle-boundness? The belief that it does is probably the most widespread of the myths. As mentioned in the previous section, flexibility can actually be enhanced if one trains properly. Years ago, weight trainers may not have done so due to ignorance of many, possibly newly discovered, factors which are involved in weight training, and thereby may have become less flexible. Had the concepts of training antagonistic muscles and the proprioceptive mechanisms such as the muscle spindles and the golgi tendon organs been understood, this situation need never have occurred.

Can weight training improve cardiovascular fitness? Again, this problem was discussed in the previous section. It is generally agreed that in order for the heart to benefit from weight training, the heart rate must be kept above 140 beats per minute for an extended period of time, generally for more than 30 minutes. While this can be accomplished in weight-training regimen, it is very difficult to do because of the intensity at which one must exercise. Further, there appears to be little gained in the vital area of stroke volume, due to the constriction of capillary blood flow in the exercised muscles. Probably the safest statement to make at this time is that weight training can be an invaluable adjunct to other systems of training which are more suited to increasing stroke volume along with maintenance of a high heart rate during exercise.

Are weight lifters dumb? The stereotype of the big, strong, lummox just off the farm comes to mind. This stereotype apparently stemmed from the formerly held belief that if one spent too much time in the gym, rather than in more scholarly pursuits, he would not become as learned as his non-weightlifting contemporaries. There is some evidence that, due to the high need-achievement found among most athletes involved in individual sports (including weight lifting), their pursuits off and on the gym floor are engaged in with success as a necessary goal. Therefore, one must conclude that weight lifters, like any other class of athletes, are at least average in intelligence, and may even experience greater levels of accomplishments than do their nonathlete contemporaries, again, possibly due to their high need for achievement. Many other psychological, parameters can be considered here as well. Athletes, for example, tend to be more affiliative, more aggressive, less-self-effacing, more managerial and less hostile than nonathletes. While these personality traits may or may not be related to their IQ or learning capacity, they do speak to the point that many of the personality traits held dear in our culture are to be found in greater abundance among our athletes.

Is weight lifting dangerous? Any competitive sport, when pursued on the championship level, can be dangerous. You are asking the body to perform at a level far above that which it is designed for. Football is the classic example, with all the broken necks, fractured fingers, and torn knees. Competitive weight lifting is no exception to this general rule. However, sport, if pursued for sports' sake or for fitness, is not necessarily dangerous. As has been discussed throughout the present chapter, weight training, when employed in the manners mentioned, actually can prevent many of the injuries common in sports. Weight training is not dangerous, and if conducted in a scientific and safe manner (e.g., using spotters while performing heavy lifts), can be the difference between getting injured or staying healthy in sports.

Do weight lifters' muscles turn to flab later in life? First of all, muscle tissue and fatty tissue are entirely different—one cannot become the other. Generally, athletes eat more during their active careers than most people, primarily due to their greater need for nutrition. Some athletes continue their eating habits even after dropping from competition, and as a result put on fat because their bodies no longer need the amount of calories they once did. Most, however, appear to remain relatively fit and trim long after their active years as athletes, probably because of reasons connected with their ego and self-image. Weight lifters are no exception to this rule. There is no reasons to believe that weight lifting, per se, contributes to obesity, and every reason to suspect otherwise.

Can one spot-reduce through weight training? There is a general adage among body builders regarding fat removal. Stated briefly, "last on, first off" or, "first on, last off." As calories are consumed in excess of the individual's daily energy requirements, fatty deposits accumulate, generally beginning around the midsection and upper hips, since these are the locations in closest proximity to the small intestines, where absorption of foodstuffs occurs. From there, deposits are made peripherally, gradually extending out to the limbs. While this course of events is an oversimplification in that one can develop fatty deposits peripherally before an enormous midsection is developed, it is nonetheless a useful guide in determining the extent to which one can reduce body fat concentrations. One cannot expect to lose fat in a localized area by exercising that area. It is the muscle tissue that is being exercised, and fat deposits are generally unaffected. Girth measurements can be reduced, however, but these reductions are probably due to the firming of underlying muscles rather than a real loss in fat. The best guide to follow in losing fat is to monitor your diet. More will be said on nutrition later.

Do women become overly muscled through weight training? Here, a value judgment is called for, regarding what constitutes feminine appearance. Only the extreme male chauvinist would lend credence to preconceived notions of femininity. The joy and exhilaration afforded the male in athletics should be, and is, available to the female as well. Weight training is an integral part of the preparatory process in most sports, and women need the benefits of such training as much as men. Further, weight training for women is an excellent method of achieving fitness for the same reasons that it is so for men. There are obvious differences in what one can expect as outcomes, however. Men have greater supplies of the hormone testosterone than do women. This hormone is responsible for the greater capacity of the male to save nitrogen, necessary in the biosynthesis of muscle protein. This greater protein synthesis is what allows men to develop tremendous musculatures, and conversely, the lack of great amounts of testosterone in women generally negates this possibility. Needless to say, this aspect of masculinity-femininity can be represented by two overlapping distributions, a fact which explains why a few women have very masculine features and why a few men have relatively feminine features. On the whole, however, the great majority of women need never worry about becoming overly muscular—it's not within their capacity to do so.

Before dropping the subject, however, one must consider what can be accomplished by women engaging in weight-training programs. Women can expect to experience the same benefits as men in every instance—it is the degree of gain which will differ. Again, this difference in degree is relative to one's position within the respective overlapping distributions.

Summary

The astute reader has, by this time, realized that there are many different ways in which the overload factor can be manipulated. Listed in Figure 2-4 are some of the more common methods. Bear in mind, however, that there should be bounds within which the lifter must operate during overload, and these bounds are governed by his specific objectives, such as size, power, or muscular endurance. An example of these delimitations is presented in Figure 2-5. Reference to the key factors in each of these areas should remain of paramount concern to the lifter, regardless of his specific objectives. That is, in training for power, tension, and speed are essential; in hypertrophy training it is variation of exercise regimen that will result in complete development; and in training for muscular endurance, one should be aware that oxygen transport and utilization are essential. Choosing the appropriate system of overload for each of these objectives will result in maximized gains in the shortest time possible. Finally, the SAID and isolation principles are vital to the efficient realization of personal objectives, and should therefore be incorporated along with appropriate overload.

---

1.   Increasing the weight being lifted

2.   Increasing the speed of movement per repetition

3.   Stricter adherence to the isolation principle

4.   Increasing the range of movement per repetition

5.   Increasing the duration of effort per repetition

6.   Increasing the number of sets and/or repetitions

7.   Minimizing the resting time between sets and/or repetitions

8.   Maximizing the activity level during rest periods

9.   Increasing the number of exercises per day

10.   Increasing the number of training sessions per day and/or week

---

Figure 2-4. Different methods of achieving overload in training. (Adapted from Morehouse & Miller, *Physiology of Exercise*, C.V. Mosby Co., Saint Louis, 1976, p. 254.)

Variable	Power	Size	Muscular Endurance
Load (% of maximum)	90-100	70-80	60-70
Duration (seconds)	5-10	30-40	90-120
Repetitions per set	Approx. 5	10-15	Approx. 40
Sets per exercise	Approx. 5	Approx. 4	Approx. 3
Rest between sets (minutes)	3-4	4-5	1-2
Speed per repetition (% of maximum)	90-100	80-90	70-80
Workouts per week	3-4	5-6	10-14

Figure 2-5. Prescribed methods of overload for power, size, and muscular endurance. (Adapted from Morehouse & Miller, *Physiology of Exercise*, C.V. Mosby Co., Saint Louis, 1976, p. 255.)

Systems of Training

Contents: *Light to Heavy System*
            Heavy to Light System
            Rest-pause System
            Compound Exercise System
            Set System
            Cheating System
            Split Routine System
            Peripheral Heart Action System
            Circuit Training System
            Interval Training
            Functional Isometrics
            Isokinetic Training
            Negative Resistance Training
            Cyclic Training Systems

Table: *3-1. Example of a Yearly Cycle*

3

In the preceding chapters, the methods of achieving muscular development and the mechanisms underlying it were discussed. Let us now consider some of the more popular *systems* of training, both those of the past as well as those currently in use. In some cases, aspects of a system may not seem to coincide with physiological principles. It may be that, in such cases, research efforts of exercise physiologists had not been available to the practitioners. In any event, such problems will be pointed out whenever possible. Bear in mind, however, that most systems have become popular because they work! Also, while many of the systems may overlap with regard to underlying principles, often it is the system's unique qualities that have rendered it useful.

A common mistake made by weight trainers, particularly physique artists, is to assume that if an exercise or system works for a champion, then it must be the best system for me. While this is certainly a possibility, it is more probable that it works for the champ only because of his greater ability or higher level of fitness. The same system may be too strenuous or too advanced with regard to the finer developmental characteristics for the beginner or intermediate level lifter.

Another common mistake made by many weight trainers is to adopt a system and apply it to all aspects of their regimen, often indiscriminately. While most systems are adaptable to an entire training regimen, there often appear to be problems, such as sticking points, staleness, or overtraining, which necessitate mixing systems. One system may work best for arm development, while another may be more suited to leg or trunk development. Only trial and error over a considerable period will resolve this problem—indeed, many lifters wallow in despair over such problems for an entire career! The truly open-minded lifters, and the lifters willing to experiment with systems are those who eventually stand a better chance of hitting upon the best combination of systems, and thereby stand a better chance of making rapid progress toward personal goals. One point remains of critical importance. That is regardless of which system or combination of systems one chooses, strict adherence to basic principles of weight training will yield the best results.

33

Yet another mistake made by the novice lifter and experienced lifter alike is the practice of keeping few or no training records. It is often asking too much for a lifter to look back on his training, often months in the past, and remember which system, how much weight, how many reps and sets, and what the training circumstances surrounding his progress were. Only complete and accurate records can allow a lifter to engage in such reflection, and only such reflection will allow a lifter to alter or modify his training regimen according to his or her specific capabilities. The final chapter of this text is devoted to maintenance of accurate training records. The wise and devoted student will do well to heed the example of the great lifters of the past and present, all of whom rely heavily upon such record keeping in establishing training regimen for themselves.

Before progressing into discussion of the various systems of weight training, it should be clear to the student who has read the preceding chapters that any system of training can be adapted to yield maximal gains in any one of the three basic areas—strength or power, hypertrophy and local muscular endurance. This is so, since it is the *method* of performing each set that largely determines an exercise's function in this regard. Bear in mind, then, throughout the following discussions, that while a particular system may be suited to development of hypertrophy, for example, the basic principles of hypertrophy training must be adhered to in implementing that system in order that the lifter will experience maximal adaptation effects.

Light to Heavy System

This training system achieved popularity among Olympic lifters during the 1930s and 1940s, and consists of progressively adding weight to a bar such that the lifter is able to perform only one repetition. The lifter begins by performing a set of 3-5 repetitions with a light weight, adds five pounds, performs 3-5 reps, adds again, and so on until failure. This procedure is followed for each of the lifter's exercises; complete recovery should follow each exercise. Three lifters work together, and a large amount of small weights are required in order that this system works effectively.

Heavy to Light System

Popularized in the early 1950s, again by Olympic weight lifters, this system is the mirror image of the light to heavy system. The lifter begins each exercise with maximum poundage, performs the given number of reps, removes five pounds, performs more reps, and so on until only the empty bar remains. Fatigue appears to be the key element in this system, as the lifter's capacity to perform the exercise diminishes with each repetition. A variation of this system is to perform each set such that the weight is reduced following each repetition. Again, three lifters are essential, as are large number of small weights.

Rest-pause System

Also called the California Set System, this system involves the lifter performing one repetition with maximal weight, resting a few seconds, performing another repetition, resting, and so on until failure. This system appears to be useful in improving strength, particularly in the learning factor.

Compound Exercise System

In this system, the critical factor is the time element. If the lifter is pressed for time to exercise, two or more individual exercises can be combined to save time. For example, rather than doing curls and presses separately, the lifter curls the weight and presses it in one motion. This system violates the important principle of isolation, since generally only the weaker movement (i.e., in this case, the curl) will benefit from overload.

Set System

By far the most popular and versatile system of weight training, the set system involves performing an exercise for a given number of repetitions, resting a minute or two, repeating, and so on for the required number of sets. This system is adaptable to practically any objective, since the sets and reps can be altered accordingly, as can the resistance, speed, rest period, or cadence. There are many variations of the set system, including the popular *super set system* and the *super multiple set system*. The super set system involves performing an exercise for one set, and following it with one set of an exercise designed to develop the antagonistic muscle(s). For example, curls followed by tricep extensions are together referred to as one super set. The super multiple set system is similar, except that the required number of sets are performed in one exercise before progressing on to the antagonist's exercise, as opposed to alternating them.

Cheating System

In the so-called cheating system, the lifter swings the weight past the weak portion of the movement, and finishes the movement in a strict fashion. This practice enables one to effectively overload the stronger portion of the movement, an area missed by exercising conventionally. For example, the curl movement, due to leverage disadvantage, is weakest near the extended position, and becomes stronger as the elbow nears 90° flexion. By using other muscles synergistically to swing the weight past the extended, weak position, far more weight can be handled in order to overload the stronger, 90° area of the movement. When used in conjunction with strict movements, this system is extremely effective in producing total muscular development.

Split Routine System

Generally, this system is employed by body builders who are engaged in developing as many muscles as possible. Since so many exercises are required to achieve total muscular development, the lifter splits his routine into two groups, and trains each group on alternate days. Typically, such grouping might include the following breakdown: Group One (Monday, Wednesday, and Friday), arms, legs, and trunk; Group Two (Tuesday, Thursday, and

Saturday), chest, shoulders, and back. The important point in this type of system is to spread the exercises out such that the same muscles are not exercised every day. A common variation of the split routine system is called the *blitz system,* where the lifter performs all of his arm exercises on one day, chest exercises the next, legs the next, and so on for the week. This system is generally used by body builders in preparation for a physique competition, and is often used in conjunction or combination with a split routine or some variation of the set system, in order to force as much size increase as possible before the contest. A further variation of the blitz system is the *hourly blitz system,* wherein the lifter blitzes one part of his/her body every hour on the hour all day. Again, this is generally used in the precontest phase, and is not a recommended system for the average athlete due to its extremely strenuous nature.

Peripheral Heart Action System

Blood shunting is the key to this system of training. The lifter performs an exercise, and follows it by an exercise for a muscle or muscle group far removed from the first, then continues on to another exercise far removed from the second, and so on until all of his exercises are performed. The theory is that by keeping the blood in constant circulation, undue fatigue will not be experienced in any given muscle, thereby facilitating recovery and ultimately general muscular development. The exercises are generally arranged in groups, called sequences. The lifter performs all of the exercises of the first sequence, repeats the same sequence three times, moves on the next sequence, repeats it three times, and so on until five sequences are performed. Each sequence consists of around five exercises for different body parts, and no exercise is repeated in subsequent sequences. There is much to be said for this system of training, especially if one's objective is overall fitness. It is an extremely tiring system, although the fatigue is not of the local variety, but rather general systemic variety. One's heart rate is generally maintained at above 140 BPM throughout the exercise session, which normally lasts for an hour or more.

Circuit Training System

In many ways related to the PHA system, this system emphasizes the time factor. A circuit consists of a group of exercises, each located at a "station." The lifter attempts to perform all of the exercises within a given "target time," gradually reducing the target time as he or she becomes more fit. For athletes engaged in a specific activity, the exercises included in the circuit should be selected according to the requirements of that activity. An infinite variety of circuits is possible, but should be constructed with basic principles in mind. Generally, this system, like the PHA system, is performed with lighter loads, and is therefore more suited to endurance development. In fact, there is much evidence to support the notion that these systems are well-suited to development of cardiovascular/cardiorespiratory function. As noted in a previous chapter, however, these claims are open to question in light of the possible inhibitory effects these systems have on the heart's stroke volume. More research is needed to clear this issue.

Interval Training

While interval training techniques have traditionally been used for endurance events in athletics, it is adaptable to weight training as well. In interval training, short bursts of activity are alternated with periods of rest for recovery. The duration and intensity of the activity and rest periods are closely monitored, and successively shorter rest periods, together with successively longer, more intense activity periods is the objective. The principle of progressive overload is served in one of five ways: (1) progressively increasing the duration of the activity interval, (2) the intensity of the activity interval, (3) decreasing the duration of the recovery interval, (4) increasing the intensity of the activity during recovery (complete rest is not advised, since some muscular activity is required for removal of lactic acid and other metabolites), and (5) increasing the repetition of the interval. Generally, one's heart rate is kept at a minimum of 150 BPM during the activity interval, and maintained at around 120 BPM during the recovery interval.

A wide variety of intervals have been devised for endurance athletes. In weight training, light weights are generally used, in a fashion similar to the PHA and circuit training techniques mentioned above.

Functional Isometrics

Functional isometrics combines, to a limited extent, qualities of both isotonic contraction (an actual shortening of the muscle takes place) and isometric contraction (static contracture against an immovable object). Initially, the lifter explosively moves the weight 2-4 inches against retaining pins, and sustains exertion against the pins in an isometric fashion for about five seconds. Theoretically, the initial isotonic phase of the exercise forces neuromuscular adaptation insofar as the movement pattern is concerned, while the isometric phase is largely concerned with intensity of effort in forcing adaptation. The harder one tries to push against the retaining pins, the more motor units are forced into action.

One of the drawbacks of purely isometric training is that one becomes stronger only at the angle he is exercising the muscle, a phenomenon presumed to be resultant of neuromuscular function. A drawback of isotonic training is that only the weakest portion of a movement can be overloaded effectively. Functional isometrics appears to be a method of reducing these drawbacks, in that only a limited range of movement is used (typically, the weakest part of a movement, called the sticking point), thereby facilitating overload without attendant neuromuscular specialization to the point where only that location in the movement is strengthened. Research is scanty at best, particularly in regard to the psychological and physiological mechanisms underlying this system's usefulness. However, if one can trust the experience of the great lifters of our time, many of whom use this system adjunctively with other systems, moderate to exceptional improvement in strength can be achieved. Because of the high intensity of effort involved in this system, it is recommended as a preseason system, to be employed for no more than a 4-6 week period. For competitive weight lifters, it is suited for precontest peaking, but not especially recommended for off-season training except for possible remedial purposes.

Isokinetic Training

Isokinetic training appears to effectively circumvent virtually all of the drawbacks of conventional systems of training. In fact, every single piece of research reviewed indicates that this system at least has the potential to equal or exceed (in some cases by a considerable margin) the development capabilities offered by isometrics or isotonics. Basically, this system employs a method of accommodating resistance—that is, the speed of movement is held constant, thereby allowing for complete overload throughout the entire range of a muscle's movement. Specialized apparatuses engineered to accomplish this speed control are used and, while generally rather expensive, are extremely adaptable to meet individual exercise requirements. One manufacturer's description of isokinetic exercise, corroborated by numerous research reports, reads as follows:

> Resistance is a function of the force applied. The isokinetic device retards the speed at which the user can move throughout a "full range of motion." The load will accommodate anything from fingertip pressure to hundreds of pounds. The user applies maximum effort and an isokinetic device automatically varies the resistance. As the muscle's tension capacity and skeletal advantage varies through the range of movement, the resistance naturally accommodates to the muscle's force transmitting capacity at every point in the range. Isokinetic constantly loads the muscles near their maximum with each repetition regardless if it is the second or tenth repetition of the exercise, and without overstressing or understressing the muscles at any point. Thus, the accommodating resistance of the exerciser correlates to the user's immediate and specific muscular capacity.*

There are tremendous advantages to such a system, to be sure. Probably the best advice at this time would be to supplement other weight-training systems with isokinetic training. Specific movement patterns related to individual sports may often be difficult to perform on such devices, therefore making it necessary to include exercises which facilitate skilled movements as well. This would be especially true for Olympic weight lifters, involved in moving the bar in specific patterns, often requiring ballistic muscular action and generation of stretch reflex, functions not capable of being reproduced isokinetically. Nonetheless, isokinetic training appears to offer the best alternative to weight training that has ever been devised. It will be interesting to observe this system's progress over the next few years, as well as the many records which promise to be broken as a direct result of isokinetically developed performance capacity.

Although background research involving methods and systems of training isokinetically is minimal, what has been done indicates that the same basic considerations with regard to repetitions, sets, resistance and cadence should be adhered to as in conventional training systems. As in other systems, the SAID, overload and isolation principles apply in isokinetics.

Negative Resistance Training

As discussed previously, isotonic contractions are of two general categories—concentric and eccentric. While concentric contractions involve a shortening of the gross muscle, as in flexing the elbow, eccentric contractions is that phase of the movement wherein the muscle is

*Mini-Gym Inc. (Printed advertising brochure), Independence, Mo., 1976, p. 3.

lengthened against resistance, as in lowering the weight after curling it. Research indicates that eccentric (or negative) movements are only about one-third as costly, from the standpoint of energy expenditure, as are concentric contractions. Since gravity is acting upon the weight being lifted in a constant amount, more muscular exertion must be used to raise the weight than to lower it. In other words, more motor units are responding in the concentric portion of the exercise than in the eccentric portion. However, if one were to use excessively large weights and perform the eccentric portion of the lift, with a partner or partners assisting in returning the weight to the starting point between each repetition, far greater numbers of motor units appear to be stimulated to respond. There is some evidence that such a system of training can yield greater strength than its concentric counterpart which uses far lighter weights. Apparently the concentric portion of a lift suffers the disadvantage of being effective only at the weakest angle of the movement, whereas the lowered weight, by controlling the speed of descent, suffers no such disadvantage. It does, however, cause severe discomfort because of the myofibrillar elements being damaged. The raking of the tiny cross bridges across one another produces friction in excessive amounts, as well as tearing of the individual elements, causing muscular soreness which lasts for several days.

The advantages offered by the negative movements are, from most reports, outweighed by the inherent disadvantages—the soreness and the difficulty involved in finding lifters capable of effectively acting as partners. Further, in light of the recently developed isokinetic theory, which overloads the entire range of movement in a concentric fashion while at the same time completely eliminating the eccentric portion, negative training appears to be of limited merit. Many physique artists, wishing to garner as much size increase as possible from their regimen, still use negative training, but generally do so with the same amount of weight as they use in the concentric phase of the exercise—in fact, they leave them together. This practice is referred to as *continuous tension* exercising, and involves lifting the weight through only a portion of the total movement without resting between repetitions. Also called *partials,* or *burns,* this system emphasizes overloading individual segments of an exercise differentially, according to which muscle is being isolated, and/or which portion of the joint action is stronger or weaker from a leverage perspective. There is much to be said for this practice, as it apparently has been very effective in yielding great gains in muscular size.

Cyclic Training Systems

All athletes need to be aware of how to get the most out of their yearly training in order to maximize their competitive efforts. However, many athletes all too often peak for a contest or meet too early in the season, and consequently are "burned out" by the time the season's end approaches. They forget that the most important meets of the season are generally at the end of the season. Consequently, a cyclic system, which necessarily differs for each sport (in fact, very possibly for each athlete) must be devised which will allow the athlete to achieve his optimal potential at the important meets, rather than at the earlier, less important ones. The principles governing cyclic training are similar for all sports, although the specific methods and systems followed may vary considerably. Generally, all athletes should divide their year into four phases: developmental, preparation, competition and recovery. A brief description of cyclic training was presented in Chapter 2.

During the *developmental period,* which lasts about four months, the athlete concentrates on skills that he or she has had difficulty with during the previous competitive season. Specific physical requirements are maximized during this period. For competitive weight lifters, it is power, while for long-distance runners it is endurance, including cardiovascular/respiratory endurance as well as local muscular endurance. During the *preparation phase,* the athlete hones his skills to a fine edge, increasing the intensity of his workouts. This phase lasts for about three months, and precedes the actual competition phase. During the *competition phase,* the athlete maintains very high intensity in all workouts, and works thoses skills and physical attributes which he or she has found to be deficient after the first two or three meets. For most sports, the competition season lasts for about four months. It is, therefore, imperative that the athlete identify beforehand those meets or contests which are of greatest importance, and attempt to peak for those. This is accomplished in the following manner. Choose the two most important meets, and train for them, regarding all other meets as practice sessions. For the less-important meets, do not cut back on workout intensity the week prior to the meet, but do so for the important ones in order that complete recovery is effected. Also, do not discontinue supportive exercises before less-important meets, but do so for important ones.

While specific requirements may vary for individuals or sports, Table 3-1, devised by a leading weight lifting expert, is illustrative of the general concept of cyclic training. The table presented is meant to be a guide for beginning Olympic weight lifters.

Table 3-1. Example of a Yearly Cycle

	Phase I	Phase II	Phase III	Phase IV
Technique	60%	40%	30%	30%
Power	20%	40%	10%	10%
Olympic lifts	10%	15%	60%	20%
Fitness	10%	5%	0%	40%

As can be observed in the above table, the *recovery phase* emphasizes total fitness and technique. In the case of the Olympic weight lifter, this fitness emphasis would relate to endurance work, while for another athlete, power might be emphasized. The principle is that one should work on overall fitness while recovering, and particularly those aspects of fitness in which he or she is generally deficient.

There appears to be little use for cyclic training in body building. The trend nowadays among physique artists is to stay in peak condition the year round, varying workouts and diet only a few weeks before each competition. It's very difficult to put on muscle mass, so most physique artists tend to keep what they have—in fact, increase it—all year. Higher reps with lighter weights are used just prior to contest time, and diet is rigidly controlled to drop as much body fat and water weight as possible. This is to expose the muscle to its greatest advantage, without excess water or fat filling the striations of the peripheral musculature. This procedure is referred to as "cutting up" and is definitely not a recommended practice for the general athlete. In fact, most physique artists admit to fatigue and lethargy after such a cutting up period. There are many misconceptions concerning athlete's diets, and these will be covered in a later chapter. For now, however, it should be fairly obvious that such a contest diet violates practically all of the principles of sound nutrition, and the physique artist would be the first to admit it. That is why he uses it only before selected contests, and for a two-week period at the most.

Specialized Exercises and Apparatuses

Contents: *Exercises for the Arms*
Exercises for Muscles of the Shoulder Joint
Exercisises for Muscles of the Shoulder Girdle
Exercises for Muscles of the Neck
Exercises for Muscles of the Trunk
Exercises for Muscles of the Hip Joint
Exercises for Muscles of the Knee Joint
Exercises for Ankle and Foot Muscles
Exercises for Muscles of the Wrist Joint and Hand
Conclusion

Figures: *Descriptive sequence photographs are presented for each of the exercises covered.*

4

This chapter catalogues many of the most widely used exercises and the apparatuses upon which or with which they are performed. The student should bear in mind that many of the exercises are highly specialized in the sense that they yield specific results. Accordingly, it remains imperative that the student adopt those exercises that suit his or her specific objectives—no athlete can do all the exercises catalogued here. The preceding chapters are therefore required reading before delving into an exercise program, for they are designed to give the student insight as to the proper methods of exercising, as well as assisting in clarifying personal objectives.

The catalog system employed in this chapter involves a basic approach. Each body part (i.e., the major joints) is discussed separately with regard to the movements each is capable of performing. The muscles which are listed are, for clarity, only the prime movers—the assistant movers, stabilizers, and synergists are not listed. If the student's training regimen must become so complex as to require consideration of these other muscles, reference to any good kinesiology text is recommended. Listed below is a brief definition of each of the terms used to describe the various movements.

Movements of the Elbow Joint

    flexion—drawing the hand toward the shoulder
    extension—straightening the arm

Movements of the Forearm (radio-ulnar joint)

    pronation—turning forearm so thumbs point forward
    supination—turning forearm so thumbs point backward

Movements of the Shoulder Joint

    flexion—raising arm forward from side
    extension—lowering arm from flexed position to side

adduction—lowering arm from sideward extension toward body
abduction—raising arm from side laterally
horizontal flexion—drawing arm across body from sideward extension
horizontal extension—moving arm from flexed position to sideward extension
inward rotation—turning arm forward (accompanies forearm pronation)
outward rotation—turning arm backward (accompanies forearm supination)

Movements of the Shoulder Girdle (Scapular Movements)

elevation—drawing shoulders upward as in shrugging
depression—drawing shoulders downward toward sides
abduction—spreading shoulders so as to broaden back
adduction—drawing shoulders together so as to pinch scapulae
upward rotation—scapulae rotate upward accommodating arm elevation above
    head
downward rotation—arms drawn against side causes scapulae to rotate downward

Movements of the Spinal Column

Cervical Spine (Neck)

flexion—chin to chest
extension—facing straight ahead (spine hyperextended when looking up)
lateral flexion—while looking straight ahead, cocking head left or right
rotation (same side)—rotation of head and shoulders toward muscle's side
rotation (opposite side)—rotation away from side muscle is located on

Thoracic and Lumbar Spine (Midtrunk and Lower Trunk)

flexion—drawing of ribs toward pelvis frontwards
extension—standing erect (bending backward is spinal hyperextension)
lateral flexion—bending sideways left or right
rotation (same side)—rotation of head and shoulders toward muscle's side
rotation (opposite side)—rotation away from side muscle is located on

Movements of the Hip Joint

flexion—drawing knees toward chest
extension—upper leg in line with pelvis and spine as in standing erect
adduction—drawing legs together from side straddle position
abduction—separating legs toward side straddle position
inward rotation—turning leg inward, as in walking pigeon-toed
outward rotation—turning legs outward, as in walking with toes pointing out

Movements of the Knee Joint

flexion—drawing heels toward buttocks
extension—straightening leg as in erect standing position
inward rotation—with knee flexed at 90°, turning toes inward
outward rotation—with knee flexed at 90°, turning toes outward

Movements of the Ankle and Foot

dorsiflexion—drawing toes toward front of leg
plantar flexion—pointing toes as in standing on toes
inversion—soles of feet facing inward (accompanies plantar flexion)
eversion—soles of feet face outward (accompanies dorsiflexion)

Exercises for the Arms (Elbow and Radio-Ulnar Joints)

Flexion. Biceps brachii, brachialis, brachioradialis

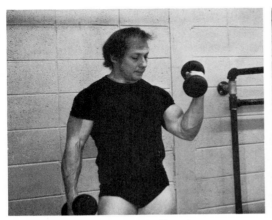

Figure 4-1. Alternate dumbell curls.

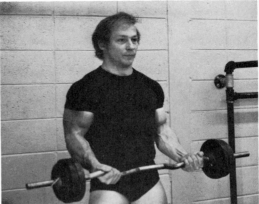

Figure 4-2. E-Z curls.

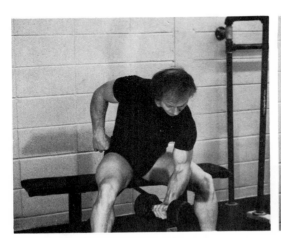

Figure 4-3. Concentration curls.

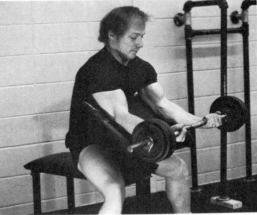

Figure 4-4. Preacher bench curls.

Extension. Triceps brachii

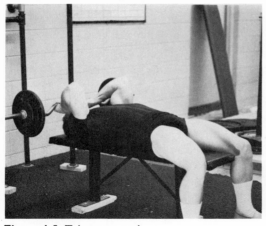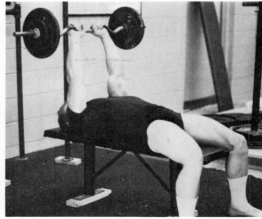

Figure 4-5. Tricep extensions.

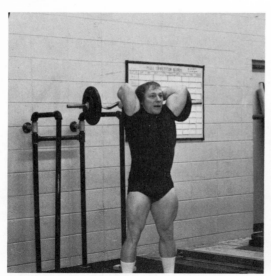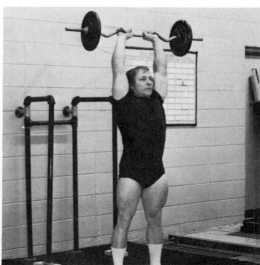

Figure 4-6. French presses.

Figure 4-7. Tricep pushdowns.

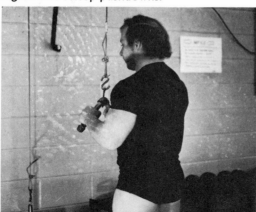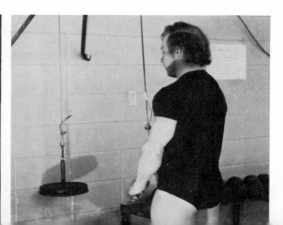

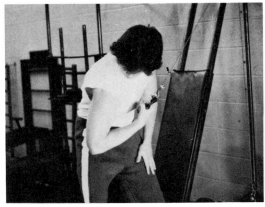

Figure 4-8. Tricep kickbacks.

Supination. Supinator   *Pronation.* Pronator quadratus

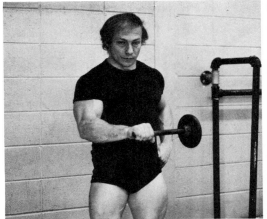

Figure 4-9. Thor's hammer.

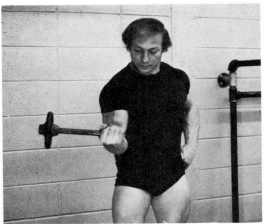

Figure 4-10. Thor's hammer.

Exercises for the Muscles of the Shoulder Joint

Flexion. Anterior deltoid, clavicular pectoralis major

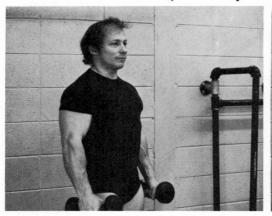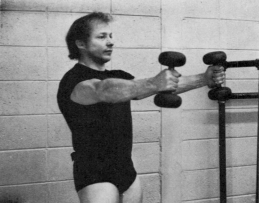

Figure 4-11. Front raises.

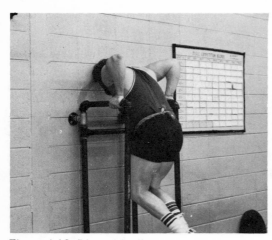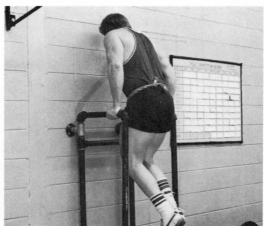

Figure 4-12. Dips with elbows out.

Figure 4-13. Incline presses.

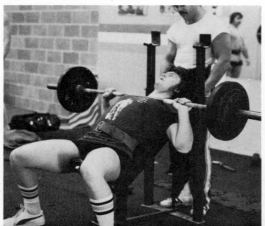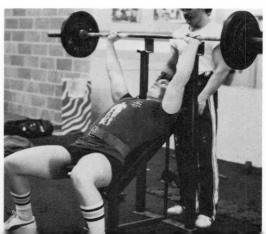

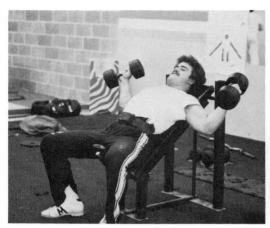
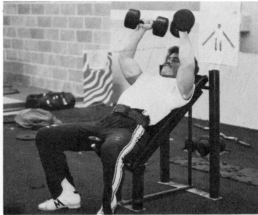

Figure 4-14. Incline flys.

Extension. Sternal pectoralis major, **Latissimus dorsi**, teres major

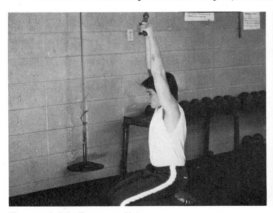
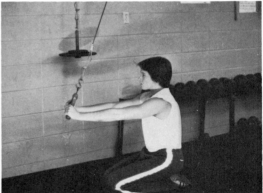

Figure 4-15. Front pulldowns.

Figure 4-16. Decline presses.

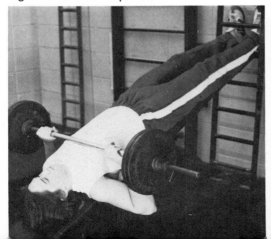
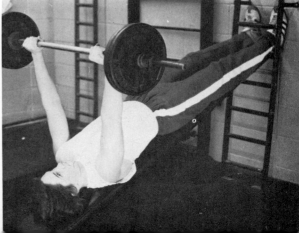

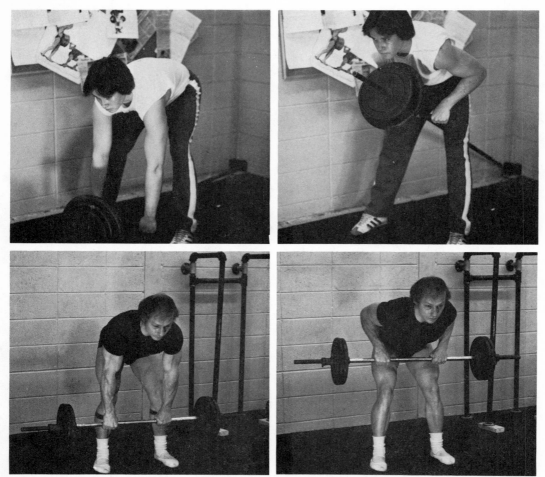

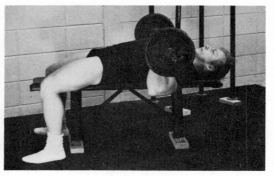

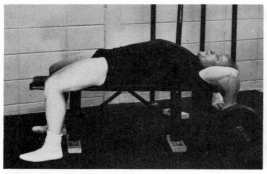

Figure 4-17. Pullovers.

Figure 4-18. Bent rows with elbows in (two methods).

Adduction. Sternal pectoralis major, Latissimus dorsi, teres major

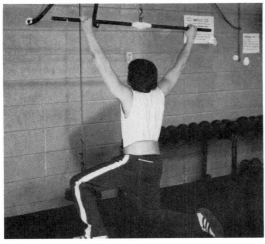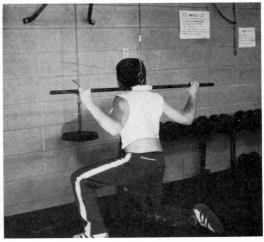

Figure 4-19. Pulldowns.

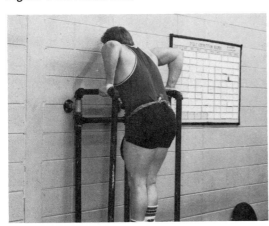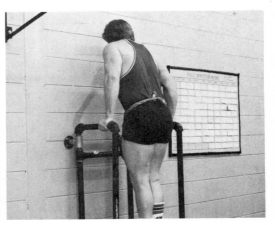

Figure 4-20. Wide grip dips.

Abduction. Middle deltoid, supraspinatus

Figure 4-21. Lateral raises.

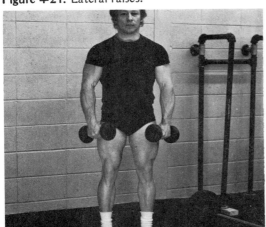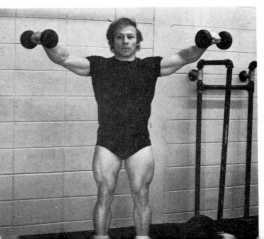

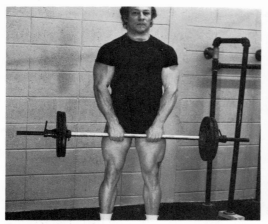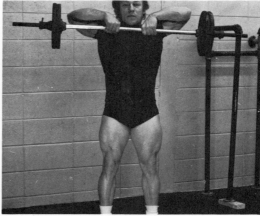

Figure 4-22. Upright rows.

Inward and Outward Rotation. The muscles involved in these movements (infraspinatus, subscapularis, and the teres major and minor) are used either as prime movers or assistant movers in other actions of the shoulder joint. No special exercises for rotation are recommended.

Horizontal Flexion. Anterior deltoid, sternal, and clavicular pectoralis.

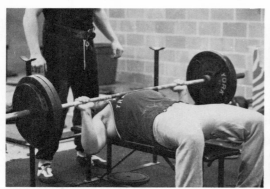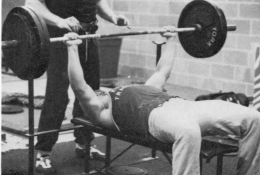

Figure 4-23. Bench press.

Figure 4-24. Supine flys.

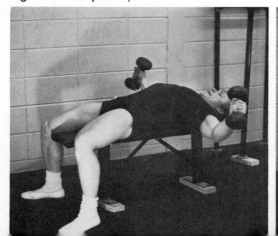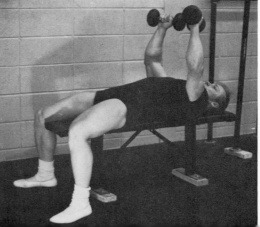

Horizontal Extension. Middle and posterior deltoid, infraspinatus, teres minor

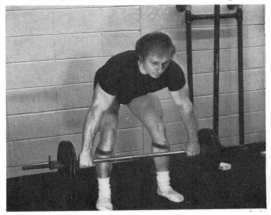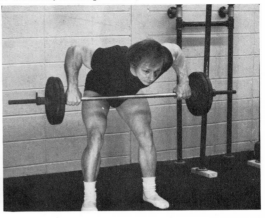

Figure 4-25. Bent rows with wide grip.

Exercises for Muscles of the Shoulder Girdle (Scapular Movements)

Elevation. Trapezius I and II, levator scapulae, rhomboids

Figure 4-26. Shrugs.

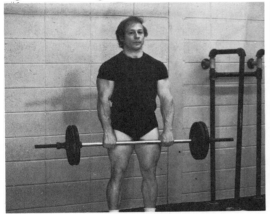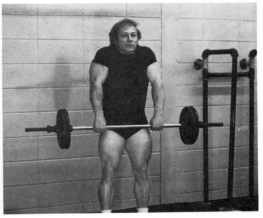

Depression. Subclavius, pectoralis minor, trapezius IV

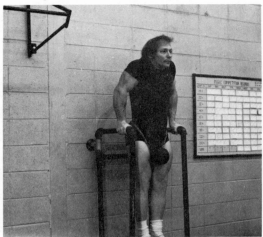
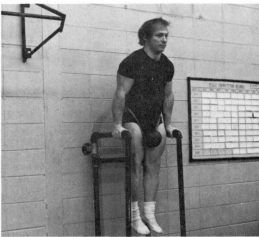

Figure 4-27. Straight arm dips.

Abduction. Pectoralis minor, serratus anterior. As in shoulder joint rotation, these muscles are involved in other movements as well as abduction, and therefore need not be exercised in pure abduction movements.

Adduction. Trapezius III, rhomboids

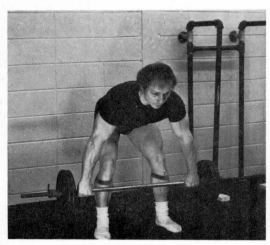
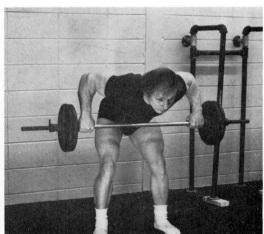

Figure 4-28. Bent rows with wide grip.

Upward Rotation. Serratus anterior, trapezius III and IV

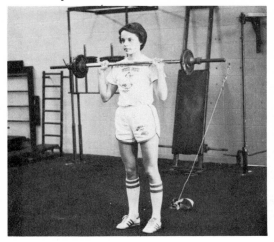 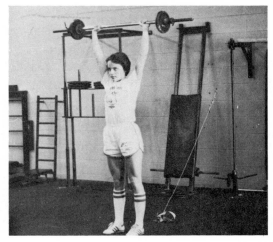

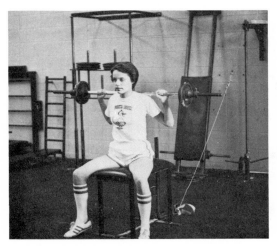 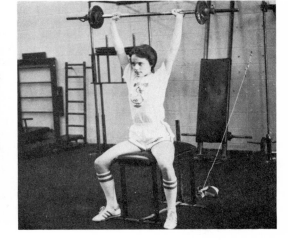

Figure 4-29. Military press—seated or standing.

Downward Rotation. Pectoralis minor, rhomboids

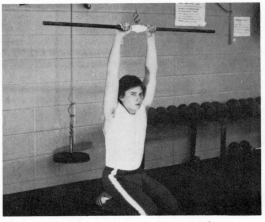 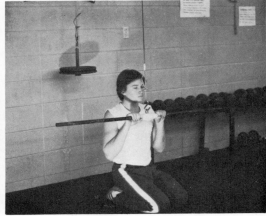

Figure 4-30. Pulldowns with narrow grip.

Exercises for Muscles of the Neck (Cervical Spine)

Flexion. Sternocleidomastoid

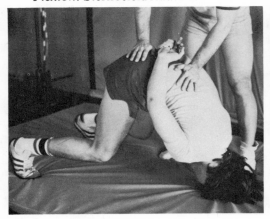 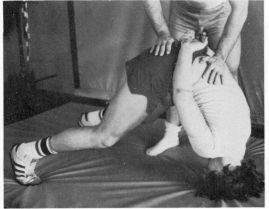

Figure 4-31. Front bridges.

Figure 4-32. Head harness.

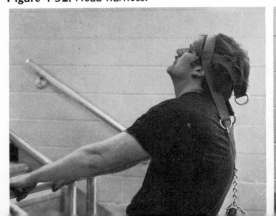 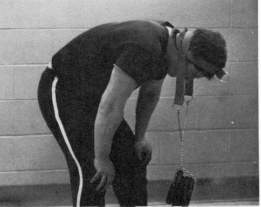

Extension. Splenius group, erector spinae group, semispinalis group, deep posterior spinal group

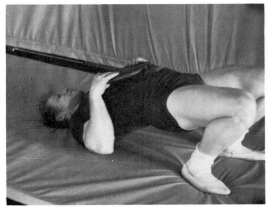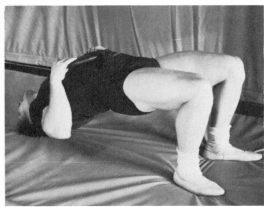

Figure 4-33. Back bridges.

Lateral Flexion. Sternocleidomastoid, scaleni group, splenius group, erector spinae group, semispinalis group, intertransversarii, multifidus

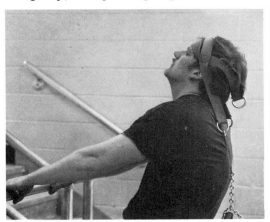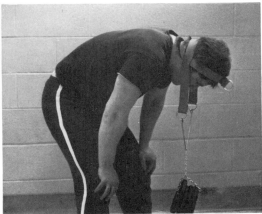

Figure 4-34. Head harness.

Rotation to Same and Opposite Sides. Splenius group, erector spinae group, semispinalis cervicus, sternocleidomastoid, rotatores, multifidus

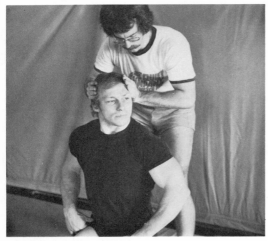

Figure 4-35. Head twists (partner).

Exercises for Muscles of the Trunk (Thoracic and Lumbar Spine)

Flexion. Rectus abdominis, external obliques, internal obliques

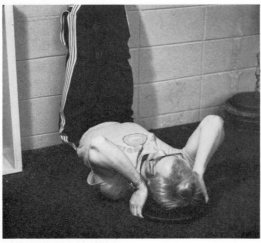 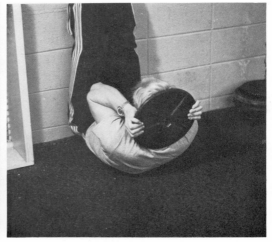

Figure 4-36. Crunchers.

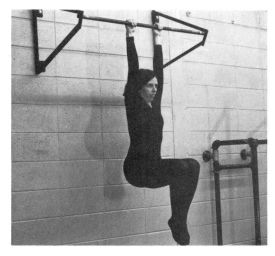

Figure 4-37. Leg raises (weighted or unweighted).

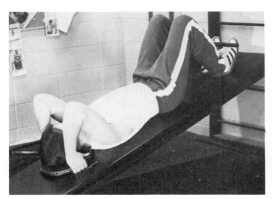 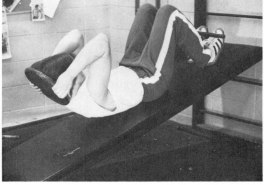

Figure 4-38. Bent leg situps.

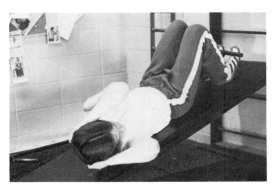 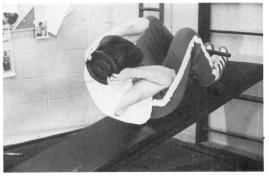

Figure 4-39. Twisted situps.

Extension. Erector spinae group, simispinalis thoracis, deep posterior spinal group

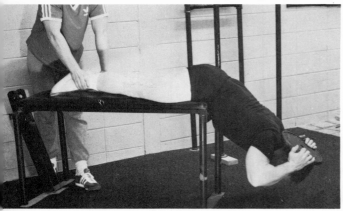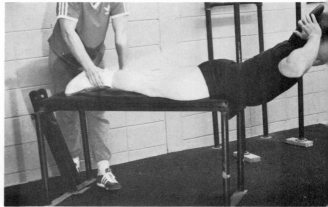

Figure 4-40. Hyperextensions.

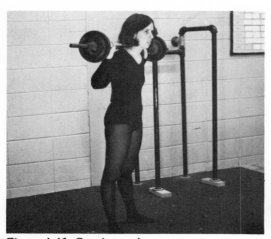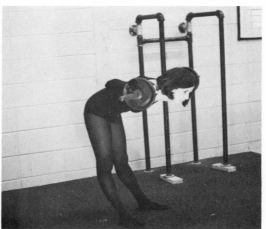

Figure 4-41. Good mornings.

Figure 4-42. Elevated pulls.

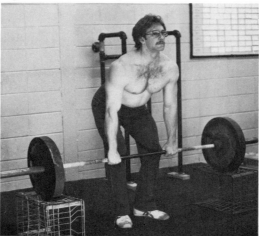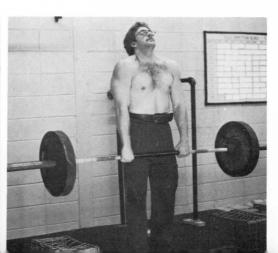

Lateral Flexion. Internal and external obliques, quadratus lumborum, erector spinae group, intertransversarii, multifidus

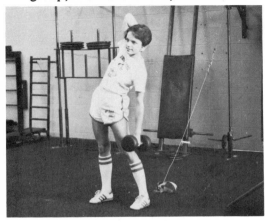

Figure 4-43. Side bends.

Rotation Same and Opposite Sides. Internal and external obliques, erector spinae group, semispinalis thoracis, rotatores, multifidus

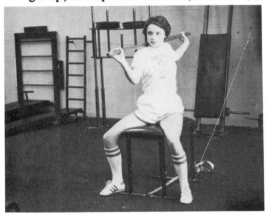

Figure 4-44. Trunk twists.

Exercises for Muscles of the Hip Joint (Buttocks and Thighs)

Flexion. Psoas, iliacus, rectus femoris, pectineus

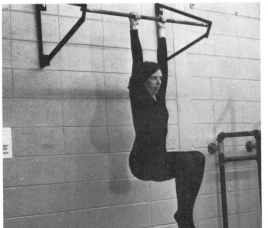

Figure 4-45. Leg raises (weighted or unweighted).

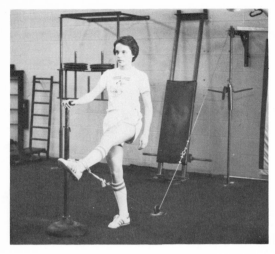

Figure 4-46. Front leg kicks (pulley).

Extension. Gleuteus maximus, bicep femoris (long head), semitendinosis, semimembranosis

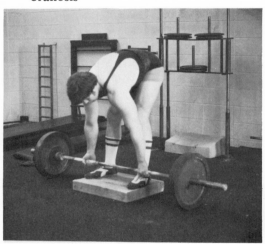

Figure 4-47. Stiff legged dead lifts.

Figure 4-48. Supine leg kicks (pulley).   **Figure 4-49.** Full squat.

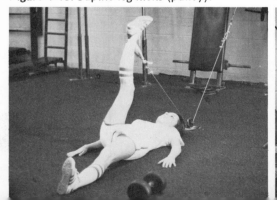

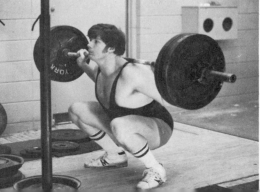

Abduction. Gleuteus medius

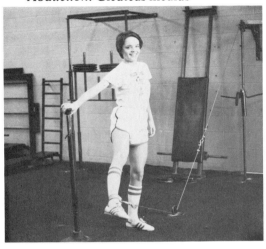

Figure 4-50. Outward leg kicks (pulley).

Adduction. Pectineus, gracilis, adductor group

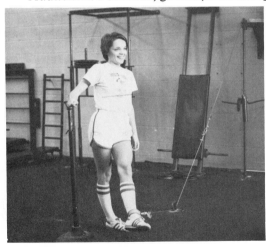

Figure 4-51. Inward side kicks (pulley).

Inward and Outward Rotation. Tensor fasciae latae, gleuteus maximus, gleuteus minimus, outward rotator group. These muscles are generally strengthened via other exercises, and consequently have no special exercises which are specifically designed for hip rotation.

Exercises for Muscles of the Knee Joint

Flexion. Semimembranosis semitendinosis, biceps femoris (hamstring group)

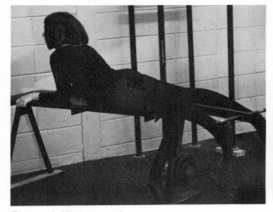
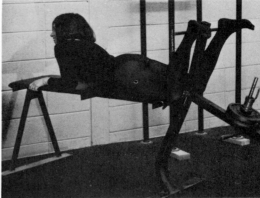

Figure 4-52. Leg curls.

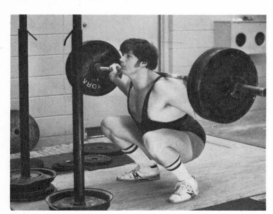

Figure 4-53. Full squat.

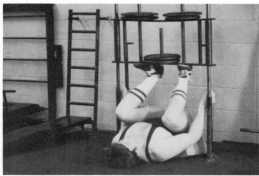
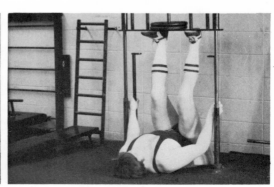

Figure 4-54. Leg presses.

Extension. Rectus femoris, vastus lateralis, vastus medialis, vastus intermedius (quadricep group)

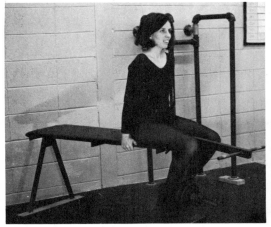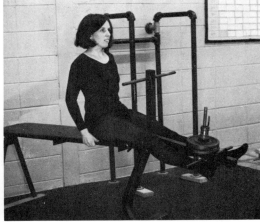

Figure 4-55. Leg extensions.

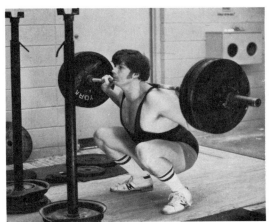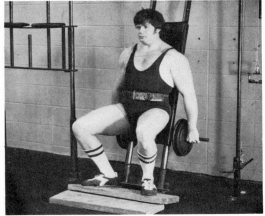

Figure 4-56. Full squat.   **Figure 4-57.** Hack squat.

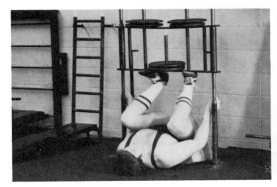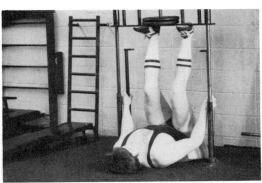

Figure 4-58. Leg presses.

Inward and Outward Rotation. Semimembranosis, semitendinosis, popliteus, biceps femoris. These muscles are generally strengthened via other exercises. Therefore, no specific exercises are recommended.

Exercises for Ankle and Foot Muscles

Dorsiflexion. Tibialis anterior, extensor digitorum longus, peroneus tertius

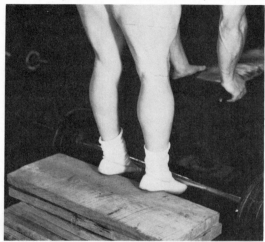

Figure 4-59. Ankle curls.

Plantar Flexion. Gastrocnemius, soleus

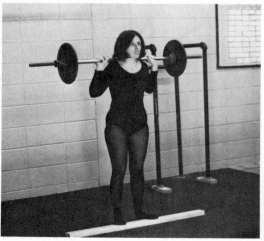 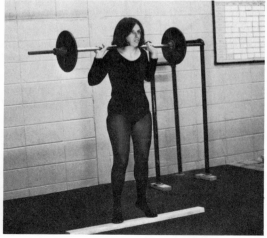

Figure 4-60. Toe raises.

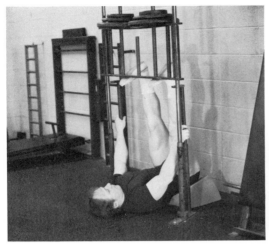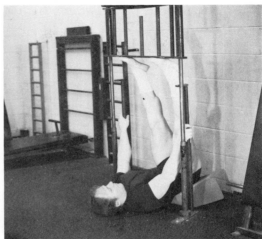

Figure 4-61. Toe presses.

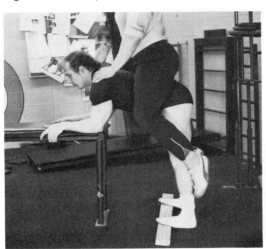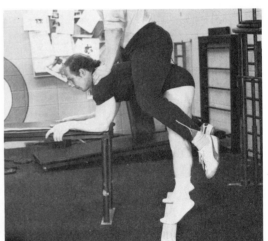

Figure 4-62. Donkey raises.

Inversion and Eversion. Tibialis anterior, tibialis posterior, extensor digitorum longus, peroneus group. These movements, and related exercises, are generally done through remediation mandates, and need not be strengthened via specialized exercises for the normal person.

Exercises for the Muscles of the Wrist Joint and Hand

Forearm development, excepting muscles involved in elbow and radio-ulnar joint actions, depends on finger and wrist exercises. This is true since most of the major muscles acting on the fingers and wrists are located in the forearm. Long tendons attach to the individual joints. Generally, simply handling weights during other exercises is sufficient to force development of these muscles. However, a few specialized exercises may be helpful:

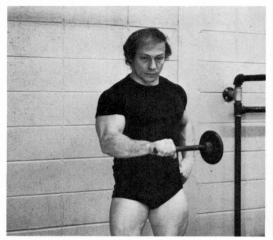 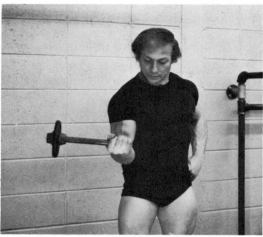

Figure 4-63. Thor's hammer.

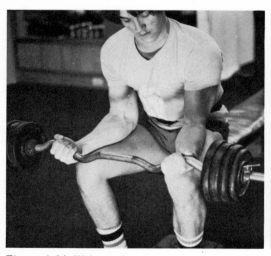 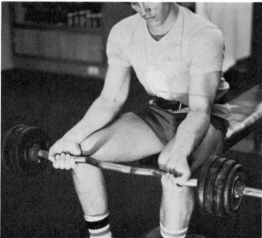

Figure 4-64. Wrist curls.

Conclusion

The student will find that each of the above exercises can be changed or adapted to fit individual needs. Many can be combined in a compound sequence. The important point to remember, regardless of one's specific goals, is that the principles of overload and isolation are absolutely essential in maximizing gains. So too is the SAID principle. The exercises catalogued here should, correspondingly, serve as a guide and model for exercise technique, but not to the exclusion of personal, sport-related needs.

One other point should be made regarding apparatus. If the student has the common problem of not being near a well-equipped facility, often he or she is forced to adapt many exercises for use with simple barbells, springs, dumbells, or other commercially available devices. Generally, this is possible, but again, attempt to adhere to the basic principles of weight training as closely as available equipment will permit.

Nutrition for Health and Athletics

5

The tremendous complexity of the biochemical mechanisms of the human body, coupled with environmental and psychological variables which are no less complex, precludes the possibility of stating in any exact terms just what constitutes a "sound" diet. There are, however, basic laws which govern energy exchange that must be used in weight gain or loss endeavors. There are also basic physiological considerations involved in determining nutritional needs, although all one can hope for in this regard is to temper them with common sense—application of known information with self-knowledge is a must in developing a sound diet. This chapter will endeavor to present basic knowledge governing weight control, nutrition for fitness as well as athletics, and will also speak to the most commonly used (and misused) food supplements and work-producing aids.

Determining Level of Underweight or Overweight

How often have you stepped on a scale and exclaimed, "Gee, I'm overweight"? Or, perhaps less frequently, "Gee, I'm underweight"? While one's weight may often indicate one's degree of leanness or lack of it, there is certainly a better indicator. One's weight says nothing of how much fat is present in comparison to one's lean body mass, and this is the critical question. Tables of average weights, such as are used by the armed forces or by insurance companies for actuarial or selection purposes, are absolutely useless, for they do not account for individual differences with regard to bone density or muscle mass. They are nothing more than a manifestation of the common misconception which has been operative in this country for a long time. The best method is to determine one's fat-free weight, and by subtraction determine how much fat is present.

There are many techniques presently in use in diagnosing obesity. *Underwater weighing* techniques make use of Archimedes' principle, wherein one's specific gravity is determined. Then, after accounting for one's residual lung volume, a corrected estimate of specific gravity is obtained. Tables have been developed to allow one to determine his/her percent of body fat from estimates of specific gravity. Underwater weighing techniques offer the best measure of percent body fat, but suffer the disadvantage of being time-consuming and requiring specialized equipment.

There are two other techniques which, while not as accurate as underwater weighing techniques, nonetheless offer fair approximations of one's percent body fat, and are much easier to administer. *Skinfold* estimates, calculated by the use of a caliper device, have been used successfully, and vary as little as ± 3% from measures derived by the underwater weighing technique. *Anthropometric* measures, which yield estimates of percent body fat varying ± 4% from underwater weighing measures are derived by measuring girths of various body parts. Both of these methods afford the fitness enthusiast or athlete information which will be invaluable in determining his/her degree of obesity, and are easy enough to use that simple weight watching should be excluded from its present level of importance. These techniques are presented in Chapter 6.

Exercise physiologists appear to be in agreement as to desired levels of body fat for average people. Ten to fourteen percent is acceptable for young men, and for women it is slightly higher, around 18%. While there are differences of opinion as to what level of body fat constitutes clinical obesity, averages for men are around 25% and for women around 35%. Many athletes have been measured at values below 5%. While recommended minimums have not been established, it should be pointed out that some fat is necessary for padding around joints, lubrication between skin and muscle, and for insulation. A safe estimate might be in the area of 5%, but this proportion may vary depending upon one's activities.

Physiology of Losing and Gaining Weight

Calorie counting is the key to gaining and losing weight. When the caloric intake exceeds the energy expenditure, a positive energy balance exists, and that energy is stored as fat. Each gram of fat produces about 9.3 kilocalories. Thus, a positive energy balance of 3,500 kilocalories will result in one pound of fat being deposited. Conversely, a negative energy balance of 3,500 kilocalories will result in one pound of fat being used as energy.

Tabled below (Table 5-1) are approximate energy requirements of various types of activities. It should be clear that, in view of the amount of activity required to "burn off" one pound of fat, something more than merely exercising is called for. Prudent dieting is the key to losing fat, and exercise is an aid. Furthermore, for reasons of psychological and social well-being, one should strive to eliminate excess body fat over a long period of time, rather than by potentially dangerous or discouraging crash diets.

Before deciding that exercise is not important, however, consider the following points. While it is neither desirable nor recommended to run the thirty-odd miles required to lose one pound of fat, running for one-half hour daily is equivalent to about a twenty-pound weight loss over a period of one year. Also, obese people (those who need to lose the weight most) do not eat more with increased activity—this is a common misconception. Their appetites actually decline with increased activity, further assisting in creating the desired negative energy balance.

Recalling from the discussion on energy sources (Chapter 1), muscular energy is derived from the breakdown of organic phosphates and glycogen. Glycogen is produced by the

Table 5-1. Energy Costs of Various Activities. Bear in mind that these figures are estimates, and vary according to sex, body weight, age, general fitness, nutrition, skill, and environmental differences, to name a few.

Activity	Kcal/Min.	Activity	Cal/Hour
Lying down resting	1.4	Sleeping	70
Standing up, inactive	1.9	Mental work (studying)	105
Driving	2.8	Bicycling (5 1/2 mph)	190
Volleyball	3.5	Gardening	295
Golf	5.0	Vigorous dancing	340
Tennis	7.1	Walking upstairs (2 mph)	590
Continuous running	10.6	Sustained running (rapid jog)	990
Swimming, 30 sec. per lap	11.5	Sustained running (fast pace)	1300
Skiing (average)	17.7	Running (18.9 mph)	9480

(Adapted from deVries, H.A., *Physiology of Exercise*, Wm. C. Brown Company Publishers, Dubuque, 1974, p. 261. Also Morehouse, L.E., and Miller, A.T., *Physiology of Exercise*, C.V. Mosby: St. Louis, 1976, p. 136-37.)

metabolic breakdown of fats, carbohydrates and protein, which are the three sources of calories. During periods of positive energy balance, fat tissue is synthesized in the liver and transported to various sites for deposit. During periods of negative energy balance, fat, generally from the last place it was deposited, is reclaimed for glycogen production. This "last on, first off" principle is the source of much discouragement among dieters, since fat is generally deposited first around the hips and midsection, where most people wish to lose it. These areas are generally the last places fat will be reclaimed from, accounting for their discouragement. Dieting prudently, and exercising regularly over a long period is the best alternative to rid oneself of these unwanted fat deposits.

Gaining weight. It should be clear that in order to gain weight (without increasing percent body fat), one must engage in some form of activity which produces muscular hypertrophy while at the same time limiting energy expenditure. The best available activity in this regard is weight training, particulars of which have been discussed in Chapters 2, 3, and 4. Many people, owing to relatively high metabolic rates, have difficulty in gaining weight. This has been found to be especially true of college students, since much psychological pressure from worrying about exams and the like contributes to tremendous levels of energy expenditure. Nervous temperament of this sort, over long periods, requires high amounts of energy. Unfortunately, there are many more people who, due primarily to lack of activity, find it very difficult to generate a negative energy balance required in weight reduction.

Losing weight. Many research endeavors of the past two decades have pointed clearly to the fact that the primary cause of obesity is inactivity—not caloric intake. While it is true that overweight people have a positive energy balance, it is also true that this positive balance stems from inactivity. Furthermore, crash diets and fasting methods are not recommended, because much of the weight lost is due to a reduction in lean body mass—not adipose tissue. Research conducted in this regard indicates that about 65% of weight lost was from muscle tissue, while only 35% was due to fat loss.

From the foregoing discussion, it can be inferred that the best alternative for losing unwanted fat is to exercise vigorously each day and to count calories as well. Overly obese people have the particular problem involving possible damage to the cardiovascular system with too strenuous an exercise program, as well as the possibility of damaging connective tissues of joints due to extreme stress. Therefore, these people should solicit the advice of a physician and train under the watchful eye of someone expert in exercise.

Recent research in methods of dieting have yielded some exciting concepts. It was found that rats gained more weight by eating their entire daily ration within two hours than did rats eating small amounts throughout the day. This method, when extended to human subjects, showed a similar trend. Obese patients fasted for 48 hours (apparently a practice designed to alter the current metabolic pattern), and then were fed 1,320 calories daily, spread over six meals. The proportions of fats, carbohydrates, and protein were 15%, 55%, and 30%, respectively. None of the patients complained of hunger, and weight losses of up to 100 pounds were reported. If any conclusion can be drawn from this research, it must be that gorging oneself at one or two meals per day is unwise, and skipping breakfast (common in this country) is discouraged. Eat more small meals.

Considerations of Sound Nutrition

Virtually all experts in nutrition recommend eating foods from a variety of sources. This practice, it is claimed, will allow the individual to obtain all the necessary vitamins, minerals, and energy sources he needs for good health. The recommended sources include vegetables, grain, dairy products, meat, and fish. In this country, as in no other, the food-fad business is booming. Faddists and food supplement companies, due to the tremendous marketability of health-giving products, have been quick to jump on the bandwagon slogan that the average American is malnourished. Using their products, which range from vitamins to wheat germ oil, bee pollen, protein, and ginseng root, they claim, will result in better health. It should be clear, however, that most of these exotic supplements are actually foods themselves, the nutritional benefits of which could be obtained far more inexpensively through other, more practical sources. Many nutritionists, exercise physiologists and FDA officials spend a lot of time and money putting down these food sources. There is nothing inherently wrong with most of them—they are, in some cases, excellent sources of many beneficial nutrients. It is clear, however, that a sound diet can be achieved in virtually countless ways and through countless sources. The safest recommendation appears to be to eat what you feel most comfortable with and can most easily afford, be the food source exotic or everyday.

The critical issue is that many Americans do indeed suffer from malnourishment—that is, a deficiency in one or more essential nutrients. A recent study involving Big Ten athletes has shown that over 35% of the athletes observed had diets deficient in vitamins A and C, and calcium. If generally health-conscious athletes' diets are deficient, it seems quite possible that the average American's diet is also.

Many people, especially athletes, cling to the hope that by supplementing their normal diets with various types of vitamin pills and other nutrients, their health, and especially their performance, will increase. They use the supplements as sort of a "hedge" against illness—an insurance policy. Many people, particularly the people in the business of selling such supplements, claim that there is nothing wrong with this practice, while others, notably FDA people, have pointed out the hazards of toxicity effects of overuse of various substances. The point is, however, that there is no scientific evidence that supplementation of a nutritionally sound diet will improve athletic performance. Those extra vitamin pills, or that heaping spoonful of wheat germ will not yield additional strength or stamina if one's diet already provides all of the essential nutrients.

Considering the importance of the big "if," it seems appropriate to supplement food intake with natural source vitamins or other nutrients during times one suspects his/her diet to be less than complete, and to disregard such a practice when one's diet is sound. Many factors are involved in determining the completeness of one's diet, and one of the most important factors is activity level.

The nature of this text precludes delving into discussion on daily requirements of various nutrients. Rather, the reader is directed to any good nutrition text wherein such lists are generally available. A brief discussion on the three basic food sources, however, seems in order, including fats, carbohydrates, and protein.

Fats, Carbohydrates, and Protein

As discussed previously, fats, carbohydrates, and protein are the three sources of one's caloric intake. Deciding on what proportion of the three sources must involve considerations of one's activity level, one's activity, and one's present percent body fat. Also, consideration must be given to identifying the best sources of the three substances.

Generally, by varying the proportion in favor of protein (i.e., reducing the amount of carbohydrate and fat in the diet), and increasing one's activity level, fat deposits will be recruited to supply the necessary energy for muscular contraction. However, should one wish to simply diet without additional energy expenditure, simply reducing the caloric intake proportionately from all three sources of calories appears appropriate. It is generally agreed that physical activity increases one's need for various nutrients, and by increasing one's intake of all foods in a balanced diet, this will be accomplished. If the activity is severe enough to stimulate muscular growth, more protein is required, but carbohydrate and fat intake should remain at a proportionate level also. Below are tables of recommended proportions derived from various sources. While similarities exist in the proportions, the differences speak to the fact that one can vary his/her diet considerably and still maintain optimal health (see Table 5-2).

The following guidelines should be adhered to in selecting food sources of fats, carbohydrates, and protein:

Fats. Saturated fats cannot combine with other substances in the body. A review of simple rules of chemistry tells one that when the molecular structure of a substance is such that all available bonds are filled, that substance becomes relatively incapable of reacting with other substances. Rancid or hydrogenated fat falls into this category. All ingested fat should be fresh and unsaturated. Animal fat is not recommended, while most vegetable fats are,

Table 5-2. Calorie Sources and Recommended Proportions

Source of Information	Percentage of Total Daily Kilocalories		
	Fat	Carbohydrate	Protein
H.A. DeVries (exercise physiologist) percentages for the average person	40	48	12
Suggested percentages for athletes in training	35	46	19
L. Morehouse and A. Miller (exercise physiologists) suggested percentages for athletes	20	65	15
S. Williams (nutritionist) athletes	35	46	19
B. Starr (strength coach for pro football team)	15*	30*	55*

*Percentages were extrapolated from other information.

providing they have not been exposed for prolonged periods (e.g., butter or margarine left out becomes saturated). Also, try to select fats rich in other essential nutrients, including vitamins, minerals, and free-fatty acids.

. While fat-free diets are not recommended since some fat is required in the metabolizing of carbohydrates, neither is a fat-rich diet. Too much fat has been linked with reduced endurance and muscular efficiency.

Carbohydrates. Of the three types of food, carbohydrates are the chief source of fuel for muscular contraction. Excellent sources of carbohydrates include most vegetables, whole grain bread, and fresh fruits, because these foods also contain many other essential nutrients. Sugar and starchy foods are generally taboo, because they offer very little in the way of additional nutrients. Aside from the obvious problem of increasing body fat proportions, high-carbohydrate diets have been linked with hypoglycemia, a condition wherein low blood sugar results from increased insulin production. Apparently, evidence is mounting to support the theory that sugar primes the pancreas to secrete more insulin, making the hypoglycemia worse. Low-carbohydrate diets, on the other hand, also appear often to be the culprit in conditions of low blood sugar. Low blood sugar causes fatigue of both the muscles and the nervous system. A fatigued nervous state results in loss of coordination and thus mechanical efficiency.

Many athletes have, in the past few years, utilized a form of glycogen supercompensation prior to an important athletic contest in an effort to increase endurance. "Glycogen loading" as it has become known as, involves a schedule similar to the following:

Days Before the Contest	Fat	Carbohydrate	Protein
7	high	none	normal
6	high	none	normal
5	high	none	normal
4	none	high	normal
3	none	high	normal
2	none	high	normal
1	none	high	none

This regimen of glycogen loading is normally accompanied by an exercise regimen which stresses high-intensity workouts early, diminishing in intensity nearer the contest. Also, the activities should be specific to the contest requirements early, diminishing to general-type exercises nearer the contest. There is much evidence indicating that such a program is beneficial for aerobic activities, but appears to be of little benefit for anaerobic-type sports. Furthermore, since it requires other than recommended allowances of the three basic foods, such a diet should be followed only before important contests—probably less than three per year. The theory behind such a practice is that by depleting one's stores of glycogen, and then replenishing them through a high-carbohydrate diet, the body adapts by overcompensation in that greater than normal levels of glycogen are stored. It should be pointed out that such a regimen may be hazardous to some athletes, particularly those who are sensitive to fluctuations in blood sugar levels, such as diabetics or prediabetics. Also, the same hazards are associated with such a diet as discussed previously regarding carbohydrate-rich or carbohydrate-deficient diets.

Protein. As with fats and carbohydrates, there are good and poor sources of protein. Proteins are composed of amino acids. Ingested proteins are broken down to their constituent amino acids during digestion, and are then resynthesized in various locations throughout the body. Of the twenty-three known amino acids, ten cannot be synthesized in the body, and must be derived from other sources. These are called the *essential* amino acids.

Diets rich in milk, eggs, and meats are high in all of the amino acids, while many vegetables lack some of the essential ones. Vegetarians must be especially careful to include a wide variety of leaves, seeds, roots, vegetables, and fruits in their diet to derive these essential amino acids. The reader is cautioned to read food labels in deciding what prepared foods are high in the essential amino acids. Unless essential amino acids are derived from other sources during the meal, the incomplete proteins are of relatively little benefit.

Aside from some of the basic considerations mentioned above, it seems unnecessary to belabor the point of good nutrition. In any event, exercise is by far of greater concern in improving athletic performance levels, especially when one's diet is reasonably sound. Simple tallying techniques will tell one which nutrients are missing from one's diet, and once identified, they should be added. Bear in mind, however, that most of the necessary nutrients for sound health are dependent upon one another, and should, therefore, be ingested together in proportionate measures. Appropriate proportions can be achieved by simple partaking in a good variety of wholesome, fresh foods. To get started on the right track, the reader is advised to purchase a pocketbook listing the various nutrients, calories and fats, carbohydrates, and proteins of various foods. Carry it with you and consult it for awhile, and soon good nutrition will be a habit.

Making Weight for Athletic Contests

For years it has been customary for athletes such as jockeys, wrestlers, weight lifters, and boxers to "sweat off" excess pounds in order to make the desired weight category. Generally, water losses of up to 5% of one's body weight can be tolerated without detrimental performance effects being noticed. Such a practice should be preceded by weeks of preparation, in that sweating out excess water disrupts the body's delicate electrolyte balance. Sodium and potassium salts are recommended as supplements to one's diet, in order that undue cramping during the contest will be prevented.

The trend nowadays appears to be for the athlete to maintain his competition weight year-round, thereby eliminating such radical procedures and their attendant side effects. Studies performed on Russian and Bulgarian weight lifters have indicated that 3.5% losses of body weight will not harm performance; losses of about ten pounds per lift were noted when the athlete was required to lose 4.5%, and about twenty pounds at 5.5%.

It should be noted that the ratio of lean body weight and fat weight may often vary for different athletes. Football linemen require some fat for greater inertia and padding from severe blows. Swimmers need some fat for insultation from heat loss in the water. Gymnasts and wrestlers need little fat, as do most weight lifters and other athletes. Fat does not contribute to increased performance, in any event; nor does excessive water weight. Close tabs on one's diet throughout the year is definitely recommended for all classes of athletes, and maintaining an equitable ratio of lean body weight to fat weight is desirable. Should the athlete find it necessary to drop water weight immediately preceding a contest, the aforementioned guidelines should be adhered to. Further, be aware that fasting for periods of time will result in debilitating losses of lean body mass to a far greater extent than of fat weight, and is therefore not recommended under any conditions.

Ergogenic Aids

Ergogenic aids, or work-producing aids, are in widespread use in practically all quarters of the athletic world. Many are banned by various sport-governing bodies due to both health and ethical considerations. Others, perhaps as dangerous or potent as many of the banned drugs and substances, are not, due to their widespread usage by the general populace. The most common of the banned ergogens include amphetamines and anabolic steroids, while the legally used substances include caffeine, nicotine, alcohol, aspartic acid, various alkalinizers, as well as many nonsubstantive procedures including music, hypnosis and loud noises. In light of health and ethical considerations, stemming from both sound research as well as the lack of sufficient research, it is recommended that the athlete engage in the use of ergogens that are neither banned nor harmful if, in fact, he must use them at all. The following discussion of the commonly used ergogens should not be construed to be supportive of their use in athletics.

Amphetamines. A known stimulant, various forms of amphetamine have been found to increase athletic performance in endurance, strength, speed, and skill. Contradictory studies indicate that, in some cases, particularly involving unskilled or novice athletes, and athletes using such stimulants for the first time, they have either no effect or, in some cases, have detrimental effects upon performance. In either case, the dangers of using the drug are well-known, and for these reasons should be avoided: (1) they are addictive—athletes addicted to amphetamines do poorly without them; (2) they block signals of impending muscular overexertion, thereby increasing the risk of serious injury; (3) vasoconstriction occurs while, at the same time, the force and rate of the heartbeat is increased; and (4) numerous cases of athletes collapsing (with, in many cases, ensuing death) from overdoses have been reported.

Anabolic steroids. Testosterone, the male hormone, has both androgenic effects as well as anabilic effects. While the androgenic component is responsible for producing masculine characteristics, the anabolic component is responsible for retention of ingested nitrogen necessary in the biosynthesis of protein. Synthetically produced anabolic steroids mimic the anabolic qualities of testosterone, thereby making it possible to recover more quickly from heavy exercise such as might be used in producing strength or hypertrophy. Since the recovery process is hastened, one can, theoretically, undergo heavy exercise more often, thereby speeding the process of muscle strength or size development. There is much contradictory evidence as to whether this drug is efficacious in its intended purpose. Many of the studies performed in this area, however, suffer from methodological flaws which tend to render them useless as sources of accurate information. Recent Eastern European studies have indicated their efficacy in the aforementioned regard, and have gone a step further by claiming that, under professional administration, they are not harmful. However, many other medical people have identified side effects that should be given consideration. They (steroids) have been found to be hepatic, carcinogenic, and responsible for undue edema, testicular shrinkage, and a host of other side effects. As with amphetamines, the traffic in steroids in the athletic community is very real, and until inexpensive and widely-administered control procedures are implemented, will remain a problem. The reader is cautioned in the strongest terms against their use. If usage is still one's intent, at least consult a physician first.

Caffeine. While a strong mental stimulant, caffeine also retards coordination. The athlete engaged in skilled movements is well-advised to stay away from coffee or tea prior to competition. Athletes engaged in activities that require little skill but high arousal have, on the other hand, noted beneficial effects in performance. However, prolonged and heavy use of coffee or tea has the debilitating effect of interfering with carbohydrate and protein metabolism, thereby offering the risk of rendering training ineffective for strength or size gains. Furthermore, since caffeine is suspected of having adverse effects on cardiovascular function, endurance athletes are well-advised to reconsider its use.

Nicotine. It is certainly unnecessary to delve into the hazards of cigarette smoking at this point in time. Objectively, however, many tobacco users appear to be relatively unaffected by smoking. There is some evidence that as high a proportion as 37.5% of young men are, however, sensitive to tobacco, and, in controlled tests of speed of movement, showed decrements in performance. It appears possible that, due to the addictive effects of prolonged use of tobacco, some men (and presumably some women also) perform better after smoking. This effect may be attributable to psychological causes, however, rather than physical. The safest recommendation is to quit—performance increases attributable to smoking are, in any case, so slight as to make any increases noted not worth the risk.

Alcohol. As tests on drivers will prove, excessive doses of alcohol are detrimental to performance and mental function. However, there is much evidence that small doses of alcohol may be ergogenic in nature, providing that the activity about to be engaged in does not require high levels of skill. One study indicated that a small dose of alcohol taken 5-10 minutes before a strength test increased performance for up to 40 minutes, but caused a performance decline thereafter. Another study involving degree of work output found that up to 240 cc of beer or brandy taken immediately or up to four hours beforehand increased the performance levels of habitual drinkers, but was detrimental to the performances of nondrinkers. The same amount taken the night before caused a marked drop in performance. There have been studies indicating that small doses of alcohol cause a decrease in O_2 debt as well as increased endurance in chilled muscles. Others show no such effects. Recent studies indicate that people who drink small doses daily over a lifetime tend to live longer than nondrinkers. While no reasons were presented for this surprising data, it appears possible that the depressant effect of the alcohol calms or lulls the user into a better night's sleep.

Whatever the case may be, as in smoking, noted increases in performance are slight at best, and the potential side effects of alcohol usage, particularly the addictive effect, warrant careful consideration on the part of the user. Furthermore, there is some evidence accumulating that excessive alcohol usage interferes with the metabolism of protein, a consideration which should be attended to by the athlete wishing to train for strength or hypertrophy.

Aspartic acid. Aspartic acid is involved in the metabolism of carbohydrates and protein. This function ultimately results in the formation of energy from carbohydrate breakdown. Studies have indicated that aspartic acid, in the form of potassium and magnesium asparates, is beneficial in offsetting fatigue, particularly in untrained subjects. Apparently, administration of aspartic acid had little effect on trained subjects. Further, little benefit was noted in the performance levels of strength athletes using aspartic acid. Since aspartic acid salts are generally considered a "food" rather than a drug, it appears that sensible use of this compound may, in some cases, be beneficial.

Alkalies. When work progresses beyond aerobic capacity, lactic acid becomes the end product of metabolism. The presence of lactic acid drastically inhibits the ability to accumulate an O_2 debt. However, if the blood is made more alkaline, lactic acid is neutralized, thereby delaying exhaustion. Numerous studies have reported increases of up to 100% in work capacity following a program of blood alkalinizing (ingestion of sodium citrate, sodium bicarbonate, and potassium citrate immediately following meals). Noted side effects, normally avoidable if the alkaline solutions are ingested after meals, include nausea, abdominal discomfort, and diarrhea. Also, alkalosis, a condition of developing too high a level of alkalinity in the blood, has been found to result in overexcitability of the nervous system, a condition which can cause muscular tetany.

Disinhibition by conditioning. While one's *true* physical capacity may be limited by physiological conditions, one's normally observed maximum physical capacity is determined by acquired inhibitions. Loud noises, music, yelling, and other methods including hypnosis have been shown to be capable of increasing performance in strength and endurance feats. Apparently, such practices have a disinhibitory effect on the organism. It is interesting that such conditioning techniques are not more widely used in athletics. In light of their seeming innocuous nature, perhaps they should be, especially considering that performance increases of from 7.4% to 26.5% have been noted through such procedures. A common anecdote is often told of the mother, in a moment of desperation, lifting a rolled-over car from her pinned child. Many such stories are confirmed, attesting to a very important conditioning component to performance. Far more research is needed in this intriguing area.

Techniques of Progress Assessment

Contents: *Simple Methods of Determining Percent Body Fat*
Skinfold method. Anthropometric method.
Determining White Versus Red Fiber Ratio
Estimating Physical Work Capacity
Test for General Fitness

6

In weight training, as in any worthwhile endeavor, efficiency in terms of time expenditure and derived benefits is desirable. Frequently, although one has arduously and meticulously adhered to basic principles such as those described in the preceding chapters, plateaus are reached, beyond which the exerciser cannot progress. Also problems of boredom, overtraining, diet, health, and injuries often tend to prohibit gains. In the interest of efficiency, reasonably complete record-keeping is recommended to all fitness enthusiasts and athletes alike. Problems are easily identified and training procedures which are contributing positively or negatively toward attainment of one's training objectives, once recorded, can be referred to without reliance on memory. Past performance levels can be related to preceding training practices to insure that future training—and subsequent performance levels—are maximized. Such objectivity is lost if memory is relied upon as the sole source of information regarding training and performance.

On the other hand, such record-keeping and measurement procedures would tend to be a hindrance, more than an aid, if they required extensive time, effort, or apparatus. There must be objectivity in records and measurements analysis, true, but elaborate equipment and time consuming methods of measurement and record-keeping are not necessary. The remainder of this chapter deals with simple, but reasonably effective and objective methods of progress assessment for the weight-training enthusiast. Also included are samples of graphs, workout logs and norms for strength, endurance, and general fitness. Periodic self-testing will give the trainee an objective gauge by which to judge his/her progress, and record-keeping will supply the reference tool necessary in adjusting one's regimen when progress stalemates.

Simple Methods of Determining Percent Body Fat

As noted in the previous chapter, estimating one's ratio of lean versus fatty weight is desirable, considering the inherent dangers of excessive obesity. Two simple methods were recommended, involving skinfold estimates and anthropometric measures, respectively.

Skinfold method. Due to inherent sex differences relative to fatty deposits, it is necessary to use separate estimating procedures for men and women. The two methods are described below. To estimate one's percent body fat by the described method, both a tape measure and a skinfold caliper are required. There are many such methods available, most of which are suitable for classroom use. The critical aspect of such techniques lies in the careful manipulation of the calipers—an experienced technician should be available to take the required readings.

$$\text{Men: Body density} = 1.1043 - 0.001327 \text{ (thigh skinfold}_{mm})$$
$$- 0.00131 \text{ (subscapular skinfold}_{mm}).$$

Once one's body density is computed, use the obtained value in determining the percentage of body fat, as follows:

$$\text{Percent body fat} = 100 \text{ (4.570/body density}_{gr/ml} - 4.142).$$
$$\text{Women: Body density} = 1.0852 - 0.0008 \text{ (suprailiac skinfold}_{mm})$$
$$- 0.0011 \text{ (thigh skinfold}_{mm}).$$

Upon determining one's body density, compute percent body fat, using the same equation listed above (men).

Anthropometric method. Again, different procedures must be used in determining percent body fat for men and women. Listed below are two methods for both men and women, each of which is easily administered. All that is required is a tape measure. Caution must be used in assuring that the tape is held at a uniform tension, and positioned according to prescribed specifications.

$$\text{Men: Lean body weight} = 94.42 + 1.082 \text{ (body weight nude}_{lbs})$$
$$- 4.15 \text{ (waist girth at umbilicus}_{inches}).$$

Then, compute percent body fat as follows:

$$\text{Percent body fat} = \frac{\text{body weight} - \text{lean body weight} \times 100}{\text{body weight}}$$

An alternative method for men is as follows:

$$\text{Fat-free weight}_{kg} = 15.10 \text{ (height}^2_{meters} \times \text{ sum of the widths of each wrist at the bistyloid locations}_m \times \text{ sum of the widths of each knee at the femoral condyles}_m \times 100)_{0.712}.$$

Convert FFW_{kg} to FFW_{lbs} by multiplying FFW_{kg} by 2.2. Then, compute percent body fat by the method employed above, in the first equation.

$$\text{Women: Lean body weight}_{kg} = 8.987 + 0.732 \text{ (weight}_{kg})$$
$$+ 3.786 \text{ (wrist diameter}_{cm})$$
$$+ 0.434 \text{ (forearm circumference}_{cm}).$$

The tape should be positioned over the widest points of the wrist and forearm, respectively, in obtaining accurate measures. Diameter is computed by dividing circumference by 3.14 (*Pi*). Convert LBW_{kg} to LBW_{lbs} and compute percent body fat as described above (men).

An alternative estimation procedure for women is as follows:

$$
\begin{aligned}
\text{Lean body weight}_{kg} = \ & 8.987 \ + \ 0.732 \ (\text{weight}_{kg}) \\
& + \ 3.786 \ (\text{wrist diameter}_{cm}) \\
& - \ 0.157 \ (\text{abdominal circumference}_{cm}) \\
& - \ 0.249 \ (\text{hip circumference}_{cm}) \\
& + \ 0.434 \ (\text{forearm circumference}_{cm}).
\end{aligned}
$$

As the reader will note, the above equation is similar to the preceding one, with the exception that two additional measures are added. The addition of these two measures makes the estimate somewhat more accurate. The abdominal circumference should be taken at the greatest bulge inferior to the umbilicus, while the hip measurement should be taken at the point where the gluteals are most prominent. Again, determine percent body fat in the same manner described in the preceding equation.

Determining White Versus Red Muscle Fiber Ratio

One might query as to the relevance of obtaining information relative to the ratio of white (fast-twitch) versus red (slow-twitch) muscle fiber he/she has. Recall (from Chapters 1 and 2) that white fiber is directly related to power and speed of movement, while red fiber is related to muscular endurance. While the total mass of white or red fiber can be changed through hypertrophy training, the number (or, ratio) of white and red fibers is an inherited trait, and cannot be changed. For one to be truly objective in assessing his/her capabilities in sport, particularly at the championship level, such information can be useful in either selecting a sport within which the chances of success will be maximized, or in the construction of a suitable training regimen designed to yield maximal benefits in one's chosen specialty.

The clinical method of determining one's white/red fiber ratio is by extracting muscle biopsies, freezing them, staining and slicing them for microscopic scrutiny. However, recent research has provided a far simpler (although somewhat limited) method. By simply determining one's vertical jump ability, an estimate of the white/red ratio can be derived. This technique may be limited, however, by the extent of prior training effect. That is, an athlete who specifically trained for white fiber development, although having a higher proportion of red fibers, may do as well or better than an untrained athlete with the opposite white/red fiber ratio. For estimating purposes, however, it appears better suited than the alternative biopsy technique. Dr. James Councilman, Indiana University's well-known swimming coach, in collaboration with Dr. David Costill, Ball State University's Director of Human Performance Laboratory, has provided the following classifications, derived from testing both track and field athletes as well as swimmers. The classifications shown are for swimmers, but similar classifications can be made for runners and other athletes.

As one can see, overlap may occur between separate areas. Obviously, many other factors, such as mechanical efficiency of lever systems, technique, and especially motivation,

Table 6-1. Vertical Jump Method of Classifying Endurance Versus Sprint
Swimmers.

Vertical jump of 9-22 inches: long distance swimmers (400-1500 meters);

Vertical jump of 20-24 inches: middistance swimmers (400-800 meters);

Vertical jump of 23-26 inches: long sprint swimmers (100-200 meters);

Vertical jump of 25-31 inches: short sprint swimmers (50-100 meters).

---

must be accounted for in applying such a classification system. The reader is urged to reread the first two chapters of this text for purposes of putting the whole matter of the significance of red/white fiber ratio into its proper perspective.

The implication of the above classification is that swimmers with a low-vertical jump have a predominance of red fiber, accounting for their lack of power and greater endurance. Conversely, swimmers with a high-vertical jumping ability have a predominance of white muscle fiber, accounting for their greater power. The important point to remember is that however motivated or however highly skilled an athlete may become, it will be exceedingly more difficult for him to successfully engage in a power event if his musculature is predominantly red fiber; and it will be equally difficult for the athlete whose muscles are mostly white fiber to succeed in endurance activities.

To determine one's vertical jump ability, stand beside a wall and mark (with chalk) the highest point of reach. Then, without stepping, running, or swinging the arms (leave the unused arm at the side), jump as high as possible and mark the highest point of reach. Simply measuring the distance between the two marks will yield one's vertical jump distance. Take the best of three attempts. Don't cheat—stepping or swinging the arms tends to invalidate the test.

Estimating Physical Work Capacity

An easily administered test for determining one's physical work capacity (PWC) is afforded by the Harvard Step Test. This test is a moderately good estimator of PWC, having an error of prediction of maximal oxygen consumption of $\pm 12.5\%$. It is based on the principle that the greater one's PWC, the greater the proportion of cardiac cost paid during exercise. In other words, the greater one's PWC, the smaller the O_2 debt to be paid during recovery.

The score, which is nothing more than an arbitrarily devised scale, should become progressively higher with training (aerobic). The following standards apply: below 50—poor; below 80—average; below 110—good; above 110—excellent. The user of this test is encouraged to complete five minutes of testing. However, should the test become so fatiguing as to be dangerous or incapacitating, stop, and apply the required heart rate measurement in the appropriate time-scale row. The specifications for testing are as follows: bench height—20 inches; 30 step-ups per minute; pulse taken at the carotid artery (right side of neck) for a 30 second time period, which extends from 1-1 1/2 minutes after test. After doing 30 step-ups per minute for five minutes, sit down, wait one minute, and count the number of times

Table 6-2. Harvard Step Test Scale

Test Time	\multicolumn{12}{c}{Total Heart Beats Taken 1-1 1/2 Minutes After Test}											
	40-44	45-49	50-54	55-59	60-64	65-69	70-74	75-79	80-84	85-89	90-94	95-99
3-3 1/2	84	75	68	62	57	53	49	46	43	41	39	37
to 4	97	87	79	72	66	61	57	53	50	47	45	42
to 4 1/2	110	98	89	82	75	70	65	61	57	54	51	48
to 5	123	110	100	91	84	77	72	68	63	60	57	54
5 min.	129	116	105	96	88	82	76	71	67	63	60	56

your heart beats in 30 seconds. Apply this number to the scale above to derive your PWC score.

Test for General Fitness

Physical Fitness, as the reader no doubt has concluded at this point in the present text, is a highly personalized matter. In Chapter 2, many of the factors that are involved in athletic prowess were discussed, and are generally the same in regard to overall fitness. However, many of these factors are specific to particular sports, to specific lifestyles and needs, and may not necessarily be desirable attributes in certain circumstances. The reader is left to decide what components of physical fitness are important to him/her, and to strive to achieve them. The following physical fitness test, then, is not a definitive test of fitness. Rather, it is meant to be a guide or reference point for the user. The test is not complete. Items such as power, agility, coordination, and related items such as balance, body composition, and posture are omitted. To obtain a true picture of one's state of fitness would require exceedingly long and tiring tests of individual attributes. The present test involves only those items deemed most commonly sought. Should testing in other areas be desired, the reader is referred to any of a number of texts available which involve such tests and measures.

The test. This test is designed to measure five attributes of physical fitness. The following directions are designed to enable you to administer the test to yourself or to another person. Read these directions carefully and observe the demonstrations given by your instructor so that you will be able to get a fair evaluation of your fitness status. The norms provided in Table 6-3 are for men only.

Muscular Strength and Endurance

Hand Grip — Isometric (norms provided)

Purpose: To measure the strength of your grip, an indicator of total body strength.
Equipment: Hand dynamometer.
Procedure: Adjust the grip to your hand size. Set maximum pointer indicator at 20 pounds (not zero). Grip dynamometer in dominant hand, squeezing it with maximum force. The arm may remain stationary or move slowly (no rapid movement

permitted), but neither arm nor instrument may touch any other part of the body or another object. Squeeze as hard as possible, relax, and squeeze again (two trials).

Scoring: The maximum number of pounds of force exerted by your squeeze will be recorded on the dial. Record to the nearest pound on your score card.

Sit-ups (norms provided)

Purpose: To measure the endurance of the abdominal muscles.
Equipment: Mats and watch.
Procedure: Lie on your back with legs straight and arms extended overhead. Knees are bent until feet can be placed flat on the mat (do not tuck heels close to buttocks). A partner kneels on floor at your feet holding down your insteps with his hands (partner should not kneel or sit on your feet, but exert enough pressure with his hands to hold feet down). On the starting signal, swing your arms forward and flex your trunk until you can touch the hands of the partner. After touching, return to the supine position, touching *both* hands to the mat. Action is repeated as many times as possible in the minute time period. Partner should move your feet during the test so as to keep the distance between the feet and buttocks relatively constant.
Scoring: Each correctly executed sit-up is counted out loud by the partner and the total number executed is recorded. Time is two minutes for men, one minute for women.

Flexed Arm Hang (no norms provided)

(Alternate Test for Women)

Purpose: To measure the endurance of the muscles in the arm and shoulder girdle.
Equipment: Horizontal bar and stop watch.
Procedure: Subject jumps and grasps the bar with his hands, palms toward face, approximately shoulder width apart. The body position is adjusted so that bar is at chin level but chin is not to be over bar or touching bar. No kicking of legs or bending knees is permitted. If the body is swinging on the bar, a partner must stop it. A stop watch is started as soon as the subject is in the correct position. The timer calls off each second of time. The subject hangs in the prescribed position as long as possible. Time stops when the top of the subject's head drops below the bar.
Scoring: A partner should note the last second called off by the timer before the head drops below the bar and record this as the score.

Weight Hold (norms provided)

Purpose: To measure the endurance of the arm and wrist muscles.
Equipment: Weight and timing devices (60 lb. barbell for men, 30 lb. barbell for women)
Procedure: Stand against wall with feet 6 inches from wall and buttocks, upper back and elbows touching wall. A partner lifts the weight to a position in front of your chest. You grasp the weight (palms up) so the elbow is bent at a 90° angle or

slightly higher. On the starting signal, your partner will release the weight. You hold it as long as possible at the 90° angle.

Scoring: When either arm drops below the 90° angle, the elapsed time is recorded to the nearest second. Maximum 2 minutes.

Push-up Test (norms provided)

Purpose: To measure the strength and endurance of the arm and shoulder extensors.

Equipment: 16-18 inch bench—women; no equipment—men.

Procedure: Assume a front leaning nest position with the hands on the floor (or bench) directly below shoulders, body straight, feet on floor. Bend elbows so body is lowered toward floor (bench) and touch chest, pushing back up to leaning position immediately with a straight body. No rest or sagging of body is permitted. Do as many as you can.

Scoring: Each time you perform one complete push-up starting in the up position, going down and back to the up position, one is scored. If your body sags or rests on the mat (at all), 1/2 push-up is scored, and after two such push-ups, the test is terminated.

Isometric Wall Sit (no norms provided)

Purpose: To measure the isometric endurance of the leg extensors (quadriceps).

Equipment: Stop watch, unobstructed wall space.

Procedure: Stand with the back and buttocks against wall. Move feet slowly away from wall, bending the knees and hips so that you slide down to a "sitting" position with the heels directly below the knees and the thighs parallel to the floor with a 90° angle at the knee and hip joint, and with the back pressed tightly against the wall (as if someone had just pulled a chair out from under you). Hold this position *without* placing the hands on the thighs as long as possible.

Scoring: Score is the time to the nearest second the position was held.

Muscular Power

Standing Broad Jump (no norms provided)

Purpose: To measure leg muscle power and body coordination.

Equipment: Mat, or floor, marked in 2 inch intervals.

Procedure: Stand behind the restraining line with toes touching, but not over line. Jump using a 2 foot takeoff and landing as far forward as possible. Take three jumps alternating with a partner.

Scoring: Record for the *best* of the three jumps the number of *inches* from the restraining line to where the heels touched the mat. Repeat the trial if the person crosses the restraining line or falls backward on landing.

Flexibility

Bend and Reach Test (norms provided)

Purpose: To measure the flexibility of the trunk and lower back.

Equipment: Bench and measuring board.

Procedure: Stand on the bench with both feet touching the supporting brace of the board. Bending at the waist with the knees straight, reach with both hands (no leaning) as far down the scale as possible. Hold the lowest point for two seconds (no bobbing).

Scoring: The lowest point on the scale that can be reached and held for two seconds is noted by a partner. Score to the nearest inch (minus above toe level, plus below this mark).

Circulatory Respiratory Endurance

Twelve Minute Run (norms provided)

Purpose: To measure circulatory, respiratory endurance.

Equipment: Measured running area and timing device.

Procedure: On a given signal, begin jogging from a marked standing point. Your instructor will call off the time each minute. A partner will count the number of laps completed. (Men—run 1 1/2 miles.)

Scoring: Record the distance covered in terms of laps and fractions of laps completed when time was stopped. (Men—time elapsed for 1 1/2 miles.)

Bench Step Test (no norms provided)

Purpose: To measure the anaerobic and short-term aerobic endurance capacity of the circulatory-respiratory system.

Equipment: Six inch step benches, stop watch.

Procedure: Stand facing the bench with a partner seated behind you. On the "Go" signal, begin stepping up onto the bench with both feet, and off the bench, i.e., up right, up left, down right, down left. Continue as rapidly as possible for two minutes.

Scoring: Score one for each time both feet are placed on top of the bench.

Table 6-3. Physical Fitness Test Norms—Men

The following norms are expressed in percentile ranks. This means that a person scoring at a given rank did as well, or better than, that percent of people who have taken this test at the completion of this course. For example, a percentile rank of 70 means one did as well or better than 70% of the students who have taken this test. These norms are based on scores recorded at the end of a one-semester conditioning course.

Percen-tile Rank	Grip (lbs.)	Sit Ups (no.)	Weight Hold (sec.)	Flexion	Twelve Minute Run (1/4 mile)	1 1/2 Mile	Fitness Rating
100	160	97	115 or above	+9	2 miles		
95	148	94	85-114	+8	—		
90	137	91	75-84	+7	—		Superior
85	130	89	70-74	+6	over 1 3/4	10:15	
80	125	88	65-69	+5	1 3/4	10:16	
75	120	85	60-64	—	—		
70	118	83		+4	—		Above
65	115	82		—	Over 1 1/2	12:00	Average
60	113	80	55-59	—	1 1/2	12:01	
55	110	79	50-54	+3	—		Average
50	106	77		—	—		
45	104	75	45-49	—	—		
40	102	74		+2	Over 1 1/4	14:30	
35	100	72	40-44	—	1 1/4	14:31	
30	98	70		—	—		Below
25	95	68		+1	Over 1	16:30	Average
20	93	66	35-39	—	1	16:31+	
15	88	64	30-34	0	—		Poor
10	83	60	25-29	−1	—		
5	75	54	20-24	−2	3/4 or under		

The remainder of this chapter is a compilation of format pages including workout logs, measurement charts, and norms for selected exercises. These exercises, for which norms are provided, should be done according to the specifications presented in Chapter 4. Do each for one maximal repetition (lRM) in strict fashion to derive the appropriate percentile ranking. Warm-up thoroughly before attempting a lRM. Also, be sure to refer to the appropriate table, as there are different tables for each body weight category. Students interested in overall fitness should strive to increase proficiency in those exercises in which they scored low. Bear in mind that these lRM scores are indicators of the involved muscles' strength, and as such should not be used for estimating other parameters such as muscular endurance or power.

The logs and measurement charts are provided as references for the trainee so that he/she can, in as efficient a manner as possible, record progress and be able to refer to prior training records to rectify/alter current training procedures for maximal benefit.

Table 6-4. 1-RM (one repetition with maximum) Strength Norms for College Men

Sit-ups: Lying on floor with heels near buttocks (knees bent), and with feet secured, place weight behind head and sit up until elbows touch knees.

Curl: Leaning against wall, feet placed about 12-15 inches away from wall, curl bar to shoulders.

Upright row: Without swinging bar, and with a close grip, pull bar to chin.

Standing press: Without back lean, press bar from shoulders to overhead position.

Bench press: Lower bar to chest, pause, and press bar overhead without arching back or moving feet.

Deep knee bend (squat): With bar on back, squat down until thighs are below parallel, then stand up.

Bent over row: Bending forward with back parallel to floor, pull bar to chest, without jerking the bar or raising the body.

Back raise: With bar on back and knees very slightly flexed, bend forward until torso is parallel with the floor, and raise back up to an erect position. This is a potentially dangerous exercise, and extreme care should be exercised when performing a 1-RM.

Standard scores: This score indicates lifters' relative positions on the normal curve, with a standard deviation of 7 points.

Percentile: This score tells the lifter what percentage of other lifters fall below him on each lift, and also the number above him.

These norms were gathered from over 3,000 college aged men after approximately ten weeks of weight training.

Norms for College Age Men in Selected Weight Exercises by R.A. Berger, 1970. Reprinted by permission of the author.

BODYWEIGHT CLASS 120-129 lbs.
1-RM

Sit-up (weight) behind head)	Curl	Upright Rowing	Standing Press	Bench Press	(Squat) Deep Knee Bend	Bent Over Rowing	Back Raise	Standard Scores	Percentile
70	107.5	120	155	170	255	185	215	100	100
65	105	117.5	150	165	245	182.5	210	95	99.9
62.5	107.5	115	145	160	235	180	205	90	99.8
60	100	112.5	140	155	225	170	200	85	99.4
57.5	97.5	110	135	150	220	165	195	80	98.4
55	95	107.5	130	145	210	157.5	190	75	96.2
52.5	92.5	105	125	140	200	150	185	70	90.3
50	90	102.5	120	135	190	140	180	65	84.2
45	85	100	115	130	180	135	175	60	75.8
42.5	82.5	95	110	125	170	127.5	170	55	64.0
40	80	90	105	120	160	120	165	50	50.0
37.5	77.5	85	100	115	150	112.5	160	45	36.0
35	75	80	95	110	140	105	155	40	24.2
30	70	77.5	90	105	130	100	150	35	15.8
27.5	67.5	75	85	100	120	90	145	30	9.7
25	65	72.5	80	95	110	95	140	25	3.8
22.5	62.5	70	75	90	100	80	135	20	11.6
20	60	68.5	70	85	95	75	130	15	.6
17.5	57.5	65	65	80	85	70	125	10	.2
15	55	62.5	60	75	75	65	120	5	.1
12.5	52.5	60	55	70	65	60	115	0	0

BODYWEIGHT CLASS 130-139 lbs.
1-RM

Sit-up (weight) behind head)	Curl	Upright Rowing	Standing Press	Bench Press	(Squat) Deep Knee Bend	Bent Over Rowing	Back Raise	Standard Scores	Percentile
70	112.5	125	165	175	265	150	220	100	100
65	110	122.5	160	170	255	145	215	95	99.9
62.5	107.5	120	155	165	245	142.5	210	90	99.8
60	105	117.5	150	160	235	140	205	85	99.4
57.5	102.5	115	145	155	230	135	185	80	98.4
55	100	112.5	140	150	220	130	195	75	96.2
52.5	97.5	110	135	145	210	125	190	70	90.3
50	95	107.5	130	140	200	120	185	65	84.2
45	90	105	125	135	190	117.5	180	60	75.8
42.5	87.5	100	120	130	180	115	175	55	64.0
40	85	95	115	125	170	110	170	50	50.0
37.5	82.5	92.5	110	120	160	105	165	45	36.0
35	80	90	105	115	150	102.5	160	40	24.2
30	75	85	100	110	140	100	155	35	15.8
27.5	72.5	80	95	105	130	95	150	30	9.7
25	70	77.5	90	100	120	90	145	25	3.8
22.5	67.5	75	85	95	110	85	140	20	1.6
20	65	72.5	80	90	105	80	135	15	.6
17.5	60	70	75	85	95	75	130	10	.2
15	57.5	67.5	70	80	85	70	125	5	.1
12.5	55	65	65	75	80	65	120	0	0

BODYWEIGHT CLASS 140-149 lbs.
1-RM

Sit-up (weight) behind head)	Curl	Upright Rowing	Standing Press	Bench Press	(Squat) Deep Knee Bend	Bent Over Rowing	Back Raise	Standard Scores	Percentile
70	117.5	130	170	185	275	205	225	100	100
65	115	127.5	165	180	270	197.5	220	95	99.9
62.5	112.5	125	160	175	260	190	215	90	99.8
60	110	122.5	155	170	250	180	210	85	99.4
57.5	107.5	120	150	165	240	175	205	80	98.4
55	105	117.5	145	160	230	167.5	200	75	96.2
52.5	102.5	115	140	155	220	160	195	70	90.3
50	100	112.5	135	150	210	150	190	65	84.2
45	95	110	130	145	200	145	185	60	75.8
42.5	92.5	107.5	125	140	190	137.5	180	55	64.0
40	90	105	120	135	180	130	175	50	50.0
37.5	87.5	102.5	115	130	170	122.5	170	45	36.0
35	85	100	110	125	160	115	165	40	24.2
30	82.5	95	105	120	150	110	160	35	15.8
27.5	80	90	100	115	140	100	155	30	9.7
25	77.5	87.5	95	110	130	95	150	25	3.8
22.5	75	85	90	105	120	90	145	20	1.6
20	72.5	82.5	85	100	115	85	140	15	.6
17.5	70	80	80	95	105	80	135	10	.2
15	67.5	77.5	75	90	100	75	130	5	.1
12.5	65	75	70	85	95	70	125	0	0

BODYWEIGHT CLASS 150-159 lbs.
1-RM

Sit-up (weight behind head)	Curl	Upright Rowing	Standing Press	Bench Press	(Squat) Deep Knee Bend	Bent Over Rowing	Back Raise	Standard Scores	Percentile
75	122.5	135	175	195	290	210	230	100	100
72.5	120	132.5	170	190	285	202.5	225	95	99.9
70	117.5	130	165	180	275	195	220	90	99.8
65	115	127.5	160	180	265	185	215	85	99.4
62.5	112.5	125	155	175	255	180	210	80	98.4
60	110	122.5	150	170	245	172.5	205	75	96.2
57.5	107.5	120	145	165	235	165	200	70	90.3
55	105	117.5	140	160	225	155	195	65	84.2
50	100	115	135	155	215	150	190	60	75.8
47.5	97.5	112.5	130	150	205	142.5	185	55	64.0
45	95	110	125	145	195	135	180	50	50.0
42.5	92.5	107.5	120	140	185	127.5	175	45	36.0
40	90	105	115	135	175	120	170	40	24.2
35	85	102.5	110	130	165	115	165	35	15.8
32.5	82.5	100	105	125	155	105	160	30	9.7
30	80.5	97.5	100	120	145	100	155	25	3.8
27.5	77.5	95	95	115	135	95	150	20	1.6
25	75	92.5	90	110	125	90	145	15	.6
20	72.5	90	85	105	120	85	140	10	.2
17.5	70	87.5	80	100	115	80	135	5	.1
15	67.5	85	75	95	110	75	130	0	0

BODYWEIGHT CLASS 160-169 lbs.
1-RM

Sit-up (weight behind head)	Curl	Upright Rowing	Standing Press	Bench Press	(Squat) Deep Knee Bend	Bent Over Rowing	Back Raise	Standard Scores	Percentile
75	125	140	180	205	305	215	235	100	100
72.5	122.5	137.5	175	200	300	207.5	230	95	99.9
70	120	135	170	195	290	200	225	90	99.8
65	117.5	132.5	165	190	280	190	220	85	99.4
62.5	115	130	160	185	270	185	215	80	98.4
60	112.5	127.5	155	180	260	177.5	210	75	96.2
57.5	110	125	150	175	250	170	205	70	90.3
55	107.5	122.5	145	170	240	160	200	65	84.2
50	105	120	140	165	230	155	195	60	75.8
47.5	102.5	117.5	135	160	220	147.5	190	55	64.0
45	100	115	130	155	210	140	185	50	50.0
42.5	97.5	112.5	125	150	200	132.5	180	45	36.0
40	95	110	120	145	190	125	175	40	24.2
35	92.5	107.5	115	140	180	120	170	35	15.8
32.5	90	105	110	135	170	110	165	30	9.7
30	87.5	102.5	105	130	160	105	160	25	3.8
27.5	85	100	100	125	150	100	155	20	1.6
25	82.5	97.5	95	120	140	95	150	115	.6
20	80	95	90	115	135	90	145	10	.2
17.5	77.5	92.5	85	110	130	85	140	5	.1
15	75	90	80	105	125	80	135	0	0

BODYWEIGHT CLASS 170-179 lbs.
1-RM

Sit-up (weight behind head)	Curl	Upright Rowing	Standing Press	Bench Press	(Squat) Deep Knee Bend	Bent Over Rowing	Back Raise	Standard Scores	Percentile
75	124	145	185	215	315	220	240	100	100
72.5	122.5	142.5	180	210	310	212.5	235	95	99.9
70	120	140	175	205	300	205	230	90	99.8
65	117.5	137.5	170	200	290	195	225	85	99.4
62.5	115	135	165	195	280	190	220	80	98.4
60	112.5	132.5	160	190	270	182.5	215	75	96.2
57.5	110	130	155	185	260	175	210	70	90.3
55	107.5	127.5	150	180	250	165	205	65	84.2
50	105	125	145	175	240	160	200	60	75.8
47.5	102.5	122.5	140	170	235	152.5	190	55	64.0
45	100	120	135	165	225	145	190	50	50.0
42.5	97.5	117.5	130	160	215	137.5	185	45	36.0
40	95	115	125	155	205	130	180	40	24.2
35	92.5	112.5	120	150	195	125	175	35	15.8
32.5	90	110	115	145	185	115	170	30	9.7
30	87.5	107.5	110	140	175	110	165	25	3.8
27.5	85	105	105	135	165	105	160	20	1.6
25	82.5	102.5	100	130	155	100	155	15	.6
20	80	100	95	125	150	95	150	10	.2
17.5	77.5	97.5	90	120	145	90	140	5	.1
15	75	95	85	115	140	85	135	5	0

BODYWEIGHT CLASS 180-189 lbs.
1-RM

Sit-up (weight behind head)	Curl	Upright Rowing	Standing Press	Bench Press	(Squat) Deep Knee Bend	Bent Over Rowing	Back Raise	Standard Scores	Percentile
75	130	150	190	225	325	225	245	100	100
72.5	127.5	147.5	185	220	320	217.5	240	95	99.9
70	125	145	180	215	310	210	235	90	99.8
65	122.5	142.5	175	210	305	200	230	85	99.4
62.5	120	140	170	205	295	195	225	80	98.4
60	117.5	137.5	165	200	285	187.5	220	75	96.2
57.5	115	135	160	195	275	180	215	70	90.3
55	112.5	132.5	155	190	265	170	210	65	84.2
50	110	130	150	185	255	165	205	60	75.8
47.5	107.5	127.5	145	180	250	157.5	200	55	64.0
45	105	125	140	175	240	150	195	50	50.0
42.5	102.5	122.5	135	170	230	142.5	190	45	36.0
40	100	120	130	165	220	135	185	40	24.2
35	97.5	117.5	125	160	210	130	180	35	15.8
32.5	95	115	120	155	200	120	175	30	9.7
30	92.5	112.5	115	150	190	115	170	25	3.8
27.5	90	110	110	145	180	110	165	20	1.6
25	87.5	107.5	105	140	170	105	160	15	.6
20	85	105	100	135	165	100	155	10	.2
17.5	82.5	102.5	95	130	155	95	150	5	.1
15	80	100	90	125	150	90	145	0	0

BODYWEIGHT CLASS 190 lbs. +
1-RM

Sit-up (weight behind head)	Curl	Upright Rowing	Standing Press	Bench Press	(Squat) Deep Knee Bend	Bent Over Rowing	Back Raise	Standard Scores	Percentile
75	135	155	195.	235	335	230	250	100	100
72.5	132.5	152.5	190	230	330	222.5	245	90	99.9
70	130	150	185	225	320	215	240	90	99.8
65	127.5	147.5	180	220	315	205	235	85	99.4
62.5	125	145	175	215	305	200	230	80	98.4
60	122.5	142.5	170	210	295	192.5	225	75	96.2
57.5	120	140	165	205	285	180	220	70	90.3
55	117.5	137.5	160	200	275	175	215	65	84.2
50	115	135	155	195	265	170	210	60	75.8
47.5	112.5	132.5	150	190	260	162.5	205	55	64.0
45	110	130	145	185	250	155	200	50	50.0
42.5	107.5	127.5	140	180	240	147.5	195	45	38.0
40	105	125	135	174	230	140	190	40	24.2
35	102.5	122.5	130	170	220	135	185	35	15.8
32.5	100	120	125	165	210	125	180	30	9.7
30	97.5	117.5	120	160	200	120	175	25	3.8
27.5	95	115	115	155	190	115	170	20	1.6
25	92.5	112.5	110	150	180	110	165	15	.6
20	90	110	105	145	175	105	160	10	.2
17.5	87.5	107.5	100	140	165	100	155	5	.1
15	85	105	95	135	155	95	150	0	0

Table 6-5. Weight Training Measurement Chart

Body Area or Measurement	Date Measurement Taken						
Weight							
Upper arm							
Forearm							
Waist							
Thigh							
Calf							
Chest							
Neck							
Harvard step test							
Body fat							

1 RM's				
1. Sit-up	lbs.	Percentile	lbs.	Percentile
2. Curl	lbs.	Percentile	lbs.	Percentile
3. Upright row	lbs.	Percentile	lbs.	Percentile
4. Standing press	lbs.	Percentile	lbs.	Percentile
5. Bench press	lbs.	Percentile	lbs.	Percentile
6. Full squat	lbs.	Percentile	lbs.	Percentile
7. Bent row	lbs.	Percentile	lbs.	Percentile
8. Back raise	lbs.	Percentile	lbs.	Percentile

Specialized test results: If special tests were used to determine proficiency at a particular sport or skill, or if overall motor ability or fitness tests were taken, describe the results of the pre- and postsemester tests here.

Table 6-6. Weekly Log of Workouts

Name: Class   Date:

System of training:

EXERCISES (in sequence)	FIRST DAY				SECOND DAY				THIRD DAY		
	Sets	Reps	Wt.		Sets	Reps.	Wt.		Sets	Reps.	Wt.

*Comments:

Routine changes made this week:

*Note: Include all events which have impinged upon your workout schedule (i.e., how you feel, late getting to bed, better lifting technique, medications, etc.). This will assist you in assessing your progress more accurately.

Bibliography

Annarino, A.A. *Developmental Conditioning for Men and Women*. St. Louis: C.V. Mosby Company, 1976.

Barrow, H.M., and McGee, R. *A Practical Approach to Measurement in Physical Education*. Philadelphia: Lea & Febiger, 1971.

Berger, R.A. "Comparison Between Resistance Load and Strength Improvement." *Research Quarterly* 33 (1962):637.

Beyer, R.A. "Comparison of Static and Dynamic Strength Increase." *Research Quarterly*. 33 (1962):329.

Chui, E.F. "Effects of Isometric and Dynamic Weight Training Exercises Upon Strength and Speed of Movement." *Research Quarterly* 35 (1964):246.

Clarke, D.H. "Adaptations in Strength and Muscular Endurance Resulting from Exercise." In *Exercise and Sport Sciences Reviews*. Vol. 1, edited by J.H. Wilmore. New York: Academic Press, 1973.

Delorme, T.L., and Watkins, A.L. "Technics of Progressive Resistance Exercise." *Archives of Physical Medicine* 29 (1948):263.

DeVries, H.A. *Physiology of Exercise*. Dubuque: Wm. C. Brown Company Publishers, 1974.

Donald, K.W. et al. "Cardiovascular Responses to Sustained (Static) Contractions." *Circulatory Research* 20 (1967):1.

Gaines, C., and Butler, G. *Pumping Iron*. New York: Simon and Schuster, 1974.

Golding, L.A. et al. "Weight, Size and Strength Unchanged with Steroids." *The Physician and Sports Medicine* 2 (1974):39.

Hettinger, T. *Physiology of Strength*. Springfield, Ill.: Chas. C. Thomas, Pub., 1961.

Jaweed, J.M. et al. "Endurance and Strengthening Exercise Adaptations: 1. Protein Changes in Skeletal Muscles." *Archives of Physical Medicine and Rehabilitation* 48 (1966):296.

Johnson, L., and O'Shea, J.P. "Anabolic Steroid: Effects on Strength Development." *Science* 164 (1969):957.

Johnson, L. et al. "Anabolic Steroid: Effects on Strength, Body Weight, Oxygen Uptake and Spermatogenesis Upon Mature Males." *Medicine and Science in Sports* 4 (1972):43.

Karpovich, P.V. *Physiology of Muscular Activity*. Philadelphia: W.B. Saunders Co., 1966.

Kiessling, K.H. et al. "Number and Size of Skeletal Muscle Mitochondria in Trained Sedentary Men." In *Coronary Heart Disease and Physical Fitness*. Edited by O.A. Larson and R.O. Malmbourg. Baltimore: University Park Press, 1971, p. 143.

MacQueen, I.J. "Recent Advances in Techniques of Progressive Resistance Exercise." *British Medical Journal* 11 (1954):1193.

Massey, B.H. et al. *Kinesiology of Weightlifting.* Dubuque: Wm. C. Brown Company Publishers, 1968.

Matthews, D.K. *Measurement in Physical Education.* Philadelphia: W.B. Saunders, 1968.

McMorris, R.O., and Elkins, E.C. "A Study of Production and Evaluation of Muscular Hypertrophy." *Archives of Physical Medicine* 35 (1951):420.

Morehouse, L.E., and Miller, A.T. *Physiology of Exercise.* St. Louis: C.V. Mosby Co., 1976.

Müller, E.A. "Influence of Training and Inactivity on Muscular Strength." *Archives of Physical Medicine and Rehabilitation* 41 (1970):449.

Nichols, B.L. et al. "Syndrome Characterized by Loss of Muscle Strength Experienced by Athletes During Intensive Training Program." *Metabolism* 21 (1972):187.

Noble, L. "Effects of Resistance Exercise on Muscle Size, A Review." *American Corrective Therapy Journal* 24 (1971):199.

O'Shea, J.P. *Scientific Principles and Methods of Strength Fitness.* Reading, Mass: Addison-Wesley Pub. Co., 1976.

———. "The Effects of an Anabolic Steroid on Dynamic Strength Levels of Weightlifters." *Nutritional Reports International* 4 (1971):363.

Pollock, M.L. et al. "Effect of Training Two Days Per Week at Different Intensities on Middle-aged Men." *Medical Science and Sports* 4 (1972):192.

Rasch, P.J. *Weight Training.* Dubuque: Wm. C. Brown Company Publishers, 1966.

Rasch, P.J., and Burke, R.K. *Kinesiology and Applied Anatomy.* Philadelphia: Lea & Febiger, 1967.

Ruff, W.K. *Physical Conditioning Through Weight Training.* Palo Alto: National Press Publications, 1966.

Shephard, R.J. "Intensity, Duration and Frequency of Exercise as Determinants of the Response to a Training Regime." *Int. Z. angew. Physiol.* 26 (1968):272.

Starr, B. *The Strongest Shall Survive.* Annapolis: Fitness Products, Ltd., 1976.

Thomas, V. *Science and Sport, How to Measure and Improve Athletic Performance.* Boston: Little, Brown and Co., 1970.

Ward, P. "The Effects of Anabolic Steroid on Strength and Lean Body Mass." *Medicine and Science in Sports* 5 (1973):277.

Williams, S.R. *Essentials of Nutrition and Diet Therapy.* St. Louis: C.V. Mosby Co., 1974.

Zinovieff, A.N. "Heavy Resistance Exercise, the Oxford Technique." *British Journal of Physical Medicine* 14 (1951):129.